T0373561

"Repairing the profound damage of early abuse, neglect, and deprivation is as infinitely complex as the healing of any injury to the human organism. In this beautifully written work, Ruth Cohn describes in spellbinding detail the multiple modalities and skills that a therapist needs to bring to the table to make this work possible. She demonstrates the need for a creative use and activation of all our senses, combined with patience, compassion, humility, and hard-earned self-knowledge. This book provides clinicians and curious consumers with a roadmap to finding both a voice and a spine. A true guide to healing."

— **Bessel A. Van der Kolk, MD,**
*president of the Trauma Research Foundation, professor of psychiatry at Boston University School of Medicine, and author of the # 1* New York Times *bestseller* The Body Keeps the Score: Brain, Mind, and Body in the Healing of Trauma

"Ruth Cohn has written a beautiful book on the neglected topic of neglect, filled with insight and compassion. I highly recommend this book to every therapist."

— **Sebern Fisher,**
*author of* Neurofeedback in the Treatment of Developmental Trauma: Calming the Fear-Driven Brain

"Ruth Cohn presents a moving account of what treating neglect is like for both the client and the therapist. Using case examples, Cohn presents elegantly how to approach the clinical complexities of neglect using an integrative approach ranging from psychodynamic principles to neurofeedback and sensorimotor therapies. This book will give hope to all who continue to persevere in reaching the restoration of the self in the aftermath of agonizing attachment wounds. A must read!"

— **Ruth Lanius, MD, PhD,**
*author of* The Impact of Early Life Trauma on Health and Disease, The Hidden Epidemic, *and* Healing the Traumatized Self: Consciousness, Neuroscience, Treatment

"In this wonderful integration of theory and compassion, Ruth Cohn brings together clinical experience and psychological curiosity grounded in neuroscience. Chock full of stories that illuminate the theory, Ruth Cohn's book makes the implicit experiences of childhood neglect tangible. More importantly, she gives us a clinical framework to effectively transform the pain people live in."

— **Deirdre Fay, MSW,**
*author of* Becoming Safely Embodied *and* Attachment-Based Yoga and Meditation for Trauma Recovery

"Ruth Cohn achieves her aim of making the psychotherapy of clinical states resulting from early neglect both fascinating and rewarding. With numerous vignettes from the wisdom of her years immersed in the psychotherapy of neglect, she illuminates the most important qualities needed by the therapist. Although this book is primarily for therapists, many patients may find their experiences mirrored in a way that promotes their understanding of how they came to their difficulties in regulating emotions, in forming secure attachments, and in having a sense of the body-based self."

**— Frank Corrigan, MD,**
*author of* The Comprehensive Resource Model: Effective Therapeutic Techniques for the Healing of Complex Trauma *and* Neurobiology and Treatment of Traumatic Dissociation: Towards an Embodied Self

# WORKING WITH THE DEVELOPMENTAL TRAUMA OF CHILDHOOD NEGLECT

This book provides psychotherapists with a multidimensional view of childhood neglect and a practical roadmap for facilitating survivors' healing.

Working from a strong base in attachment theory, esteemed clinician Ruth Cohn explores ways therapists can recognize the signs of childhood neglect, provides recommendations for understanding lasting effects that can persist into adulthood, and lays out strategies for helping clients maximize therapeutic outcomes. Along with extensive clinical material, chapters introduce skills that therapists can develop and hone, such as the ability to recognize and discern non-verbal attempts at communication. They also provide an array of resources and evidence-based treatment modalities that therapists can use in session.

*Working with the Developmental Trauma of Childhood Neglect* is an essential book for any mental health professional working with survivors of childhood trauma.

**Ruth Cohn, MFT,** practices psychotherapy and sex therapy and specializes in work with survivors of childhood trauma and neglect. She is also the author of *Coming Home to Passion: Restoring Loving Sexuality in Couples with Histories of Childhood Trauma and Neglect.*

# WORKING WITH THE DEVELOPMENTAL TRAUMA OF CHILDHOOD NEGLECT

## USING PSYCHOTHERAPY AND ATTACHMENT THEORY TECHNIQUES IN CLINICAL PRACTICE

**Ruth Cohn**

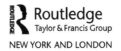

Routledge
Taylor & Francis Group

NEW YORK AND LONDON

First published 2022
by Routledge
605 Third Avenue, New York, NY 10158

and by Routledge
2 Park Square, Milton Park, Abingdon, Oxon, OX14 4RN

*Routledge is an imprint of the Taylor & Francis Group, an informa business*

© 2022 Taylor & Francis

The right of Ruth Cohn to be identified as author of this work has been asserted by her in accordance with sections 77 and 78 of the Copyright, Designs and Patents Act 1988.

All rights reserved. No part of this book may be reprinted or reproduced or utilised in any form or by any electronic, mechanical, or other means, now known or hereafter invented, including photocopying and recording, or in any information storage or retrieval system, without permission in writing from the publishers.

**Trademark notice:** Product or corporate names may be trademarks or registered trademarks, and are used only for identification and explanation without intent to infringe.

*Library of Congress Cataloging-in-Publication Data*
Names: Cohn, Ruth, 1955- author.
Title: Working with the developmental trauma of childhood neglect: using psychotherapy and attachment theory techniques in clinical practice/Ruth Cohn.
Description: New York, NY: Routledge, 2022. | Includes bibliographical references and index.
Identifiers: LCCN 2021007952 (print) | LCCN 2021007953 (ebook) | ISBN 9780367472474 (hardback) | ISBN 9780367467777 (paperback) | ISBN 9781003034407 (ebook)
Subjects: LCSH: Psychic trauma in children–Treatment. | Psychological child abuse. | Abused children–Rehabilitation. | Psychotherapy.
Classification: LCC RJ506.P66 C64 2022 (print) | LCC RJ506.P66 (ebook) | DDC 618.92/8914–dc23
LC record available at https://lccn.loc.gov/2021007952
LC ebook record available at https://lccn.loc.gov/2021007953

ISBN: 978-0-367-47247-4 (hbk)
ISBN: 978-0-367-46777-7 (pbk)
ISBN: 978-1-003-03440-7 (ebk)

Typeset in New Baskerville
by KnowledgeWorks Global Ltd.

*To Joan Cole, my first and best teacher about attachment.*

*And to Michael Lewin, my first teacher about neglect, and my best teacher about love.*

# Contents

# Acknowledgments

It definitely takes a team to write a book, and I have been blessed with a winning team. First of all, I want to recognize and thank my clients who were not only generous but also enthusiastic about sharing our story. You know who you are; Gina Ogden and Waverly Fitzgerald, who gently shepherded me to Routledge before quietly slipping away into the next world, and Anna Moore who from the first moment after I'd been delivered welcomed me to Routledge with kindness; my esteemed and trusted teachers, who enlightened, inspired and led me: Frank Corrigan, Ruth Lanius, Sebern Fisher, who is really part angel, Gavin Webber, the "CheeseMan" who kept me calm, and Bessel van der Kolk, who has been my steady GPS for going on 40 years (long before you knew me!) and never took me off course; my beloved sisters, Becki and Barbara, who handled all the complicated family matters during a particularly trying year, an incredible support for my writing; and most of all, my husband Michael, who with undying presence, has graciously shared the house since I suddenly found myself working from home, provided often needed tech and other practical support; handled the household and sick dogs, and lovingly endured a year of dreaded neglect.

Thank you all.

# Chapter 1

# Ancestral Roots

I discovered and became compelled by the developmental trauma of neglect almost by chance. I entered the field of psychotherapy in the 1980s when psychological trauma was barely making its entrance as a sub-field. PTSD was named and newly entered the Diagnostic and Statistical Manual (DSM) in 1980, largely in response to the symptom picture of the returning war veterans from Viet Nam. I grew up with the horror of that war flashing on the TV screen daily, and that was compelling enough. When sexual abuse and domestic violence against women and children came increasingly into public awareness, and the sequelae and symptoms of these traumatic experiences garnered the PTSD diagnosis as well, the nascent field called to me as an area of early specialization. I was even more drawn to it as I was the child of two survivors of the Nazi Holocaust, and had my own share of trauma, both personal and vicarious. In those days, there was not yet a literature or much training for how to treat trauma.

I soon came to hone in on work with adult survivors of childhood sexual abuse, primarily women. I offered individual and later group therapy for the women, and for 15 years had two ongoing women's survivor groups, learning much by the seat of my pants. The area of greatest pain and distress for the women invariably centered on relationship, and that was the worst of what brought them to my door (although flashbacks, nightmares and the numerous variations of suffering and dysregulation that made a living hell of their lives, were certainly significant as well). I also found that many of them were in, often longstanding, partnerships. Many complained that their partners "did not understand" or failed to support their healing process. I thought perhaps an additional way I could intervene might be by offering trauma education to partners of sexual abuse survivors, to help expand their support network. Thus emerged my first one-day workshop for male partners of survivors of childhood sexual abuse.

In that first workshop, eight men eagerly, if somewhat nervously, crowded into my office. They were of many stripes, some blue collar and others highly successful professionals. But they all seemed oddly similar. When asked about themselves, they responded by talking at length about the partner. When asked about their own story, there was "no story." They said "*nothing* happened to me." There was something ghostlike about them; their actual existence seemed to be uncertain. Yet, in the world they were highly competent and adaptive. One built houses, from scratch; one was a surgeon; one a renowned professor and author, an electrician. All had plenty beside their names. It was in the interpersonal world that they became vapid and invisible.

Trauma and its healing are consuming. As any of us who have worked with it, can attest, the survivor's entire brain and body are reset in the direction of threat and terror. Recovery is rarely quick and it is virtually diagnostic that for quite some time there is little attention for much else. What kind of person would partner, and persist long years, with someone whose interest and attention were so meager, who is engrossed and overwhelmed by pain and fear? What sort of childhood would prepare and train them to endure that kind of solitude in a partnership? These questions evolved into my interest in what I came to understand as neglect.

That first workshop day was a watershed for all of us. I did gently press them to talk about themselves. The day became lively and by the end of the day they wanted to continue meeting, and asked for an ongoing group. We continued meeting, largely intact for many years. When I began to complain that I was getting too old to work so late into the evenings, they protested. "We will pay more, we'll meet less often, but please keep it going." They were learning so much about connection from their relationships with each other. And they were the living laboratory where my nascent study of neglect began.

Starting out, I was flying somewhat blind. The trauma treatment I was steeped in, did not seem to apply to them. Clients with incident or "shock" trauma have "hyper-aroused" nervous systems, meaning they live in a chronic state of fight or flight. The freeze or numbing response, which is the one I learned about more in depth later, I would find to be more applicable to neglect. Initially, I was not sure what neglect survivors needed in the way of their own treatment.

A number of important theoretical, biological and even sociological influences have been essential in evolving my ideas about treatment for neglect ever since. I want to be sure to acknowledge, validate, connect the elements and guard against appearing to "re-invent the wheel." I do not have to reach far to recall them. We never really work alone even though solitude can create an illusion of self-sufficiency. Both the experience of neglect, and our culture of "rugged individualism" relentlessly re-enforce that myth.

## ATTACHMENT THEORY

Most significantly, attachment theory has a tremendous influence on my thinking, with its emphasis on the profound impact of relationship and relationship dynamics on psychological, emotional, social and physical development.

The British psychologist John Bowlby and his assistant Mary Ainsworth created the initial framework for attachment theory, beginning in the 1930s and 40s. The elegant theory, as the reader may know, works from the premise that our first relationships with primary caregivers, provide the template for all subsequent relationships, and the tenaciously repetitive nature of relationship patterns. Left to themselves these patterns persist through the lifespan.

Bowlby identified four main attachment styles. The first and most favorable of course, is the *securely attached*, where the parents' consistency and presence provide predictability, and a ready supply of what the infant needs to physically thrive, and also feel comfortable and safe. Of course, there is no perfect caregiver, but this child develops with a reasonable expectation of receiving a consistent supply of focused attention, gratification and protection, which contribute to the unfolding experience of having value and a sense of self that reflects that.

When the parents' presence and care are intermittent or unpredictable, the child lives in a chronic state of uncertainty, not knowing if and when they can hope to be taken care of, in general not knowing what to expect. The result is a gnawing and consuming anxiety, and later confusion about what this unpredictability means, and what it means about them. This is what Bowlby called the *anxious ambivalent* style. In the absence of a consistent, watchful eye, the child is unprotected, and vulnerable to harm, which will make for still more anxiety. This anxiety follows them through their relationship lives, making trust and calm elusive at best, and often more like a minefield.

The last-added *disorganized* style is characterized by what Berkeley attachment expert Mary Main described as the "dilemma without solution." This dilemma is that the source of comfort and the source of terror are the same person. So, the child is caught in the terrible bind between reaching toward and recoiling from that person, which results in an inability to act, or "freeze" response. My client, Lisa had such a history. Her mother at times exhibited doting attention, even appearing to favor her over her two siblings; at other times fits of fierce and painful violence; and at still other times was completely absent. During the desolate absences was when Lisa was victimized and sexually abused by others. As a young adult, she was intermittently anxious or numb; and desperately lonely, while finding relationship an impossibly unsafe gamble. After our first session, Lisa experienced a bout of what she described as paralysis. She could not get out of bed for a week. Meeting a new potential caregiver, reaching out for comfort, activated the age-old terror of danger. Then she was racked by shame. Struggling with both overt trauma and neglect, the exquisitely bright and attractive young woman perennially lamented "what is *wrong* with me?"

Bowlby's *avoidant* style is what I found most accurately describes most of our neglect clients. I object to the terminology as it can imply intentionality on the part of the child, which is hardly the case. This child's experience is primarily neglect. The parent is pretty reliably *not* present, and the child feels forgotten, abandoned or in one way or another not seen and known.

The mothers of these infants were particularly striking in that "they expressed an aversion to physical contact when their infants sought it, and expressed little emotion during interactions with them … [they] were insensitive to their infants' timing cues" and again, "seemed to dislike close physical contact with their infants."

The extreme includes physical neglect, where food, clothing, shelter and essential health care for whatever reason, are not furnished. But often in insidious cases, the parents might be in body at least, right there. Neglect resulting from parental narcissism is not uncommon. It might even include intrusiveness, but attention to what the child feels and cares about, what they need, in effect who they *are*, is bitterly lacking. The child is left alone far too much, and some of the essential developmental experiences of the parent-child interaction do not occur.

The default, of necessity, is self-reliance, and what can appear to be a "calm" indifference to others. However, the avoidant child is not really calm at all, as evidenced in the subsequent attachment research of Mary Ainsworth.

Ainsworth, an associate of Bowlby's, later established herself as a developmental psychologist in her own right. She is best known for her research known as the "strange situation." In this study, Ainsworth orchestrated a brief sequence of interactions where she observed young toddlers in four discrete interactions: when the mother left the room; when a stranger entered and approached the child; when the stranger left the room; and when the mother returned. The series was filmed, the intent being to study the reactions to separation and reunion of the different attachment styles. In my generation, we all saw the films in graduate school, and the images from those grainy old black-and-whites remain vivid and not infrequently return to my mind's eye.

About the avoidantly attached, the research showed:

> An infant classified as 'Avoidant' … will usually engage with the toys in the presence of the caregiver. The infant is unlikely to show affective sharing (e.g. smiling or showing toys to the caregiver) before the first separation …. Upon separation the infant is unlikely to be distressed …. The infant with an avoidant relationship tends to treat the stranger in much the same way as she does the caregiver, and in some cases the infant is actually more responsive with the stranger. Upon reunion with the caregiver, the avoidant infant shows signs of ignoring, turning away or moving past the caregiver rather than approaching. If picked up the avoidant infant will make no effort to maintain the contact.

I remember the poignancy of seeing the apparently self-contained little person playing quietly in the corner looking oblivious or unbothered as others came and went. Other later research on psychophysiology has consistently shown that beneath this seemingly placid little exterior, heart rate, skin conductance and EEG (electrical activity in the brain), all markers of hyperarousal/anxiety, shoot high when the caregiver leaves the room.

Of course, our adult clients don't remember their infancies. However, when I find myself visited by the images from the scratchy old movies, I don't dismiss them. I quietly notice them. When the time might be right, I might ask clients what they know about what was going on in their parents' lives when they were infants, or how old they were when a younger sibling was born. Sometimes I say nothing. In some cases, interventions including recounting aloud the description of the image in the videos are powerful. Since their first appearance in the 1970s, the research has been repeated many times, and the films, both the originals and subsequent versions are readily and freely available, and well worth watching.

Particularly painful, is the data in Attachment Theory about the mother's rejection of the physical body of the child, and of physical contact. Shame, self-hatred or at best, dramatic disconnection from the body are all things I often sadly see in these clients. Sexual and eating dysregulations are not uncommon.

Much as the theory describes, these clients are fiercely or desperately self-reliant and self-sufficient; highly sensitive to rejection and loss, and ambivalent about relationship. They more often do remember from later in childhood, that the mother was absent, distracted, narcissistic, somehow disabled or simply not interested. And these children must do for themselves. So they learn to do it all, expect that, and think little of it. It becomes their "ambient air," their "normal," their default mode, and to lesser or greater degrees, something to defend and protect.

Like the mother or the stranger in the videos, I found that indifference about the therapist; or therapist as an interchangeable part, or not necessarily distinguishable from another therapist or another person may persist for quite a while with these clients. One individual being unique or special to another may be a foreign concept, certainly (but not only) a therapist. They may think of therapy as the work of "fixing" something that is "broken," certainly not about a relationship. And of course, therapy is a different, and in some ways, odd relationship arrangement. They may precipitously leave therapy without closure, with no thought that the therapist would miss anything but the money. A therapist who needs acknowledgment or validation from the client will have a very difficult time, at least for a while.

These are extreme characterizations, and certainly not the only things we see, but attachment theory taught me to view such patterns in the light of early relationship templates. Being profoundly unseen and not known creates a dehumanizing norm, for both self and other.

## A DIP INTO PSYCHOANALYTIC THEORY: "PROJECTIVE IDENTIFICATION"

Early in my work with neglect clients, I was shocked and alarmed to discover that it could be easy to "become" that mother. I learned quickly that "projective identification" is a powerful way that clients have of communicating to us what they have no words for, and/or little if any awareness of.

In terms of communication, **projective identification** is a **means** by which the infant can feel what he/she is feeling. The infant cannot describe his feelings in words for the mother; instead, he/she induces those feelings in her.

This is of course an oversimplified distillation of one aspect of Thomas Ogden's complex interpretation of the concept. For our purposes, I would simply substitute the word "client" for infant, therapist for mother, and add possibly "behaviors" to feelings induced in the other. Being mindful of the possibility is an extremely important aspect of our toolkit. When working with people who are often acutely unaware of, or ill equipped to tell their own story, we therapists must be attentive and able to bear "impostor-like" and even repugnant feelings and behaviors that are not typically our own.

I learned this the excruciatingly hard way! Highly uncharacteristically I might forget an appointment or to return a call; a payment, or something important the client had told me. The most nightmarish, horrifying mistakes a therapist like me could imagine. Once I was incredulous to learn, I had fallen asleep. The client said with a laugh, "you fell asleep! It was only for a few seconds." He was clearly much less rattled than I was. And his reaction was similarly part of the story. He was communicating to me how utterly forgettable he had always been, but perhaps not quite consciously felt. He continued with whatever he had been talking about, appeared to promptly forget about it, and it never came up again in the several subsequent years he worked with me. Thankfully things like this have happened only rarely, and not in a long time, as I learned to be aware of this phenomenon. And because it has only happened with these clients, I consider it noteworthy. Due to his isolation, this extremely bright, literate and talented man was out of touch, unable to feel and verbalize the personal and interpersonal. I learned not only to be scrupulously attuned to "listen" very attentively to *them; but perhaps even more*, to my own inner experience, so that I could learn about what they did not consciously know and were unable to simply tell me. And preferably learning it without failing them again. This means paying the utmost attention to oneself.


**NEUROSCIENCE**

Because of my special interest in trauma, I had the good fortune to become challenged by the workings of the brain, early in my career. Bessel van der Kolk, arguably the "Father of the Modern Trauma Field" introduced research about aberrations in brain function incited by "overwhelming experience" well before anyone else was talking about brain function, with the possible exception of Daniel Amen, the first practitioner to recommend and offer neuroimaging or brain scans as part of his treatment. Amen was famous for saying, "We are the only professionals who don't even look at the organ we treat." Van der Kolk began to recognize and study the ways that "overwhelming experience" hijacked and dysregulated brain function. Traumatic stimuli to the brain, nervous system and body were greater than what the brain was equipped to process in its customary way. The advent of neuroimaging technology, and the newfound ability to observe the living brain, heralded what came to be called "the Decade of the Brain," in the 1990s, and brain research arrived at last on the mental health scene. I was proud that the still young and small subfield of trauma was in the vanguard of interest and the study of how the brain, and subsequently the nervous system, and body are dysregulated and thrown dramatically off kilter by traumatic experience, becoming both the stage for symptomatology and access routes for treatment.

Allan Schore, another important influence on this thinking, wrote a very dense, brilliant, neuroscience-based book called *Affect Regulation and the Origin of the Self* which, although it was a challenging read, had a profound influence on my thinking. In a nutshell,

Schore teaches that the infant brain develops in resonance with the brain of the mother, right hemisphere to right hemisphere, primarily through the gaze. In the case of neglect, of course, this vital function has clearly failed.

Shame being very much about rejection, hiding and also being/feeling unworthy is a ready default. Our neglected clients often wonder or struggle about how much shame they feel. The experience of being unseen beginning so early is like ambient air to them. Often eye contact is uncomfortable, even painful to them, foreign and absent. I can remember early on feeling annoyed by the complete lack of eye contact with one new client. I felt disconnected, even disrespected. I did not understand then that it was a missing experience being communicated to me. And it was also an expression of the gulf of distance between this woman and her inner world, and of course anyone else's. The most fundamental means of contact was alien, even threatening to her. I worked with her for years, and it was a phenomenal help to her when I began to practice Neurofeedback and used direct brain training devices in addition to our relationship to in effect teach contact to her profoundly lonely nervous system. She is not unique, but rather she was one of my first teachers. More will be said about working with the brain-centered approaches in psychotherapy below.

Again, the mirroring function, the most essential way a child comes to know who he/she is, has failed, right from the start. So this client is hard pressed, and left alone, to construct an identity, which is likely to be brittle at best. In turn, as we begin to try and introduce the mirroring function to an adult, it may be unpleasant, mistrusted or met with anger or contempt. Or simply rejected. However, when it begins to land and be received, the magic begins.

Once van der Kolk and Schore directed me to the brain, it became an enduring and endless pursuit. There is so much to learn that is of use. It was a natural step to study and practice brain approaches to work with these clients. Especially as such methodologies may in some ways be more "comfortable" for them as the focus is not overtly on the relationship with the therapist; and also, there is no pressure to remember or talk about their histories, which they often can't or do not want to.

Schore also got me very interested in the general function of the right hemisphere. So much emotion, color, tone and energy reside there. Experts in brain laterality such as Iain McGilchrist have commanded my attention and study, as does understanding better, what the impact is of an under-stimulated right hemisphere. Finally, trauma theory taught us about implicit and explicit memory.

Explicit memory is like a written recipe, it is narrative describing discrete and concrete, sequential autobiographical events. And explicit memory is often what is sorely lacking in the child of neglect; or it is distorted, fragmented or partial.

Implicit memory, is the residual emotion, the "felt sense" that something is familiar; behavior or symptoms that tell a story that is not verbally, cognitively or visually, consciously known. It is the memory that is not available or recognizable as memory. It is when like Proust, we are transported by a sensory experience, that we may not be able to readily place. As we work with the child of neglect, we must listen and observe with our whole body, to learn about what is unknown or missing.

As the Decade of the Brain proceeded, along with the research of the still small trauma subfield, trauma researchers began to notice that a category of children and adults did not tidily qualify for the PTSD diagnosis. They might be unable to check the boxes for flashbacks and nightmares; for example, the diagnosis as it was written was too "narrow," ignoring this population, and leaving them to slip through the cracks. Ruptured early attachments, abandonment and a host of *missing* essential experiences could overwhelm the nervous system in similar ways. But these children and adults did not meet the criteria for treatment.

Pockets of the trauma subfield did describe "Big T" and "small t" trauma in a soft or informal way. Big T connoted incident or "shock" trauma; and small t included the less overt, visible and dramatic experiences, which were assumed to be less injurious. These designations never entered formal diagnostic literature, and looking ahead we can see how by the very nomenclature, neglect would be the step-child, demeaned to a lower valence.

## FROM THE ACE STUDY OF 1995–1997 TO "DTD"

Another influence on me was ACE (Adverse Childhood Experience) Study. In the years 1995–1997, Kaiser Permanente Medical Group undertook a now-famous large-scale research project in which 17,000 members were surveyed about "Adverse Childhood

Experiences," which were then correlated to health and behavior. By now, 25 years later, these data have reached and penetrated mainstream awareness. But some 20 years ago, trauma researchers like Ruth Lanius and others were making the connections between childhood experiences besides overt sexual and physical abuses, that perpetrated profound traumatic effects, including mental and physical health and behavior. Such adverse experiences might include witnessing violence, living in war and natural disaster circumstances, poverty, parental illness or substance abuse and neglect. The lens of trauma began widening, and advancing toward much more prominently including neglect.

Renowned trauma neuroscientist, researcher and clinician Ruth Lanius wrote eloquently about this in 2010, including neuroimaging in her correlation of adverse experience to somatic symptoms. It is only relatively recently that both therapists and the public have awakened to the ACE study and its findings. We now more definitively know that this other category of experiences similarly overwhelms the brain and nervous system, and I might add at least as much. It is certainly pertinent to some of the social justice issues that are finally becoming more difficult to ignore. Often the visuals of dramatic brain scans from her studies flash through my mind as I sit with a client and feel the ways in which their bodies and the apparent rhythms of their "arousal" levels strive to tell the story that is not cognitively known.

As we entered the 21st century a group of determined trauma researchers attempted to include a code for what came to be called "Developmental Trauma" into the 2013 revision of the DSM. Their intention was to create a diagnostic category that would include and dignify this large and more quietly suffering population, and that insurance companies would honor. Large numbers of children would finally become eligible for help and care. Clearly, these adverse experiences, occurring in childhood and often very early in childhood, have an impact on brain and body that can disrupt development, and if left untreated, their entire future life trajectory.

Although researchers carried out extensive field trials with undeniable results, they failed. Developmental trauma, or DTD as we came to call it was not adopted into the psychological-psychiatric "Big Book," the DSM. As of this writing, Developmental trauma still has not formally penetrated broader professional (or public) awareness and is not yet standard graduate school training for therapists, so children of neglect are largely in the shadows, under the radar and most therapists lack the training to identify or help them. And because they themselves are so accustomed to being "invisible" these clients tend not to be "squeaky wheels" and often think "nothing happened to me" which is precisely the problem.

We in the trauma subfield continue to use the term DTD, and efforts to advance acceptance soldier on. Slowly, it is hoped, neglect is making its way into larger, more generalized awareness.


## MY PERSONAL JOURNEY

Like many of us in this field, our own experience is a tremendous impetus to both understand what happened and to discover what heals. I have been asked whether a neglect history is "training" for a career in psychothcrapy, or psychotherapy with these clients. I have not seen data on this, but it is a worthy question. I know my own history makes it far easier for me to see neglect, and to empathize. Although my "Big T" history was undeniable, the injuries of omission remained invisible and mysterious. My keen sensitivity to clients that I came to identify as children of neglect, raised the question of why I seemed so acutely attuned to these experiences. And the more I understood about myself, the better I was able to understand them. An adaptive feedback loop that I am sure is not news to the reader!

My mother, initially raised by nannies in a cold, emotionless Northern German family, saw all the perfect order of her home violently upended when Nazi soldiers stormed in. She was soon sitting alone, on the Kindertransport, a train that carried children to safety outside the increasingly Nazi dominated country. Thankfully she was spared the death camps, making her one of the survivors whose developmental trauma might be minimized or even denied. I never learned too much of her story, but she always reminded us to kiss everyone goodbye before leaving the house, because you may never see them again. We always dutifully did.

The war ended in 1945. I was born in 1955, and she already had a toddler, my older sister, by then. By the time I was two, my mother was about to give birth to her third child. Her own trauma was not only untreated but quite fresh. Treated it never was.

She married my father very quickly after meeting him, not terribly long after arriving in the United States. Both of them worked hard in this new country that accepted them as immigrants, to make a living and also learn how to live harmoniously in a stunningly foreign culture. My father was not only severely traumatized, but very driven. It was not long after their marriage, that besides being adamant about rapidly replacing the six million by quickly having a family, he was desperate to put the past behind him and create a completely new life. There was no time, no room for feeling. Very soon he was working at least two jobs while going to school full time in New York City. And although he was devoted to my mother, he did not have time for her. He was busy making up for lost time, for not finishing high school, and for the myriad ordinary experiences of youth that so many of our traumatized clients grieve about missing out on. He was determined to go to college and he did, ultimately earning a Master's from Stanford.

With respect to suffering, my father had a corner on the market. Besides being a "50's wife," still expected to fulfill a traditional woman's role, my mother remained pretty invisible until she died, a full 20 years before my father did. It was then that he sat catatonic on the couch and cried for two years. By then I had been in the trauma field long enough to suspect, he was not only grieving the loss of our mom but also, finally, the traumatic loss of his own mother when he was 12.

I remember always feeling that both my parents had terrible pain and I really had no right to exist, except for perhaps to find any ways I could to help them. That is what I undertook. So, was my childhood experience training for a career in psychotherapy with an emphasis on trauma and neglect? Well, perhaps yes. It is seldom, however, so simple. And again, there is no data about the larger question about this, as far as I know, long story short, I am no stranger to invisibility, and that is an undeniable influence.

From the experience of a long in-depth individual therapy, I can vouch for the centerpiece of healing from neglect, being the consistent and reliable presence of a caring mirror in the therapeutic relationship. Being seen, known, understood and remembered are the deepest and most developmentally salient missing experiences of neglect. Attachment theory is perhaps the most profound of my "external" influences. Interestingly, Bowlby died on my mother's birthday in 1990.

That being said, I am wholeheartedly committed to all of the other modalities and access routes that I present in this book, and all have been tested and found essential in my personal trenches, as well as in the therapy room. Nonetheless, however, as profound and powerful as all the other modalities absolutely are, the consistent, present and mirroring other, is the most essential ingredient of all. I hope this personal aspect does not make me less credible.

I have heard it said that therapists dislike neglect clients. That is not my experience at all. They can be challenging primarily because they are so averse to need, that they may be help-rejecting, oppositional and even appearing "disrespectful." They may insist that the therapy is "not helping," or appear to "know it all already." Because in many cases the crumbs of recognition that they did get were from care-taking, some may be solicitous and "good" even to the point of apparent saccharine inauthenticity. The therapist must be patient and gentle. In spite of all this, for me it has been rare to feel dislike or impatience.

What can make these clients challenging can be their sympathy and devotion to the neglectful parent(s). Although Lisa was incredulous at some of the ways her mother was completely oblivious to the horrors that were happening to Lisa under their very roof, and even when she could not help but know, she was still able to turn a blind eye, not to mention sometimes adding her own rage and violence against the tiny child. Still, Lisa was haunted by the stories of her mother's childhood, much as I was by my father's. Sympathy for her mother stopped her. So, most of the time the default to self-blame for her difficulties was a much more reliable (and ego syntonic) explanation. In a one-person world, the child is responsible for everything.

For me what is the single most challenging of all, is that lacking the experience of an attentive and present other, the survivor of neglect may themselves lack the ability for presence and contact, resulting in a yawning vacuum between us. They may not realize that when asked about themselves, their other-directed and caretaking focus has them talking primarily about whoever the important other might be, thinking they were talking about their feelings. I have often first been able to identify a neglect survivor by my own weighty sleepiness or God forbid, boredom, which is ordinarily quite foreign to me; and the seemingly interminable creep of the therapy hour, also uncharacteristic for me. That disconnection or contactless-ness, first noticeable in my own feeling state, may be a first, and often most reliable, indicator that a new client is a child of neglect. It took me a while and a measure of self-flagellation to learn this. Happily, however, it is also one of the most noticeable changes and indicators of progress and healing as the client works through the desolation of a solitary history. And it is a steady reminder to us of the vital import of our scrupulous, attentive and interested presence with them. Nonetheless, if it is unpleasant or challenging to rely on one's own inner experience to guide the psychotherapy, it will be difficult or even distasteful work.

Neglect clients may initially balk at the designation "child of neglect" especially if their neglect was at the hands of a narcissistic mother whom they experienced as wildly intrusive and demanding. They are more aware of feeling completely dominated and smothered, and far less aware of how utterly unknown and lacking in emotional understanding or mirroring they have been. With the Avoidant Attachment style, anger, shame, attentional problems and depression are common complaints. Correlating these experiences to childhood may be a hard sell at first.

I am inclined to use the term "self-reliant" because in our culture that is actually viewed as a strength, and so does not offend but even "compliments" them. Often, they are desperate for relief, not knowing what is "wrong." They may feel helpless and hopeless, and often that is their most familiar experience of the interpersonal world. Many are very high functioning and well paid in the larger context, so again their distress goes unnoticed as they look so good on the outside. We certainly don't want to replicate that!

Good consultation with a consultant knowledgeable about neglect is essential, as is a consultant able to guide the therapist through the wash of internal states that come with the territory. When our clients experience being truly seen, heard and understood is when they begin to open, unfold, bloom and take to the therapy. This is no small feat.

To me this is a fascinating and rewarding journey. I hope to convey that and encourage the passion and motivation that I feel to bring this vast population out of the darkness. Recognizing the various challenges, I will attempt to address both what to *do* clinically, how to work with *one's own feelings* and how to bring the language of neglect into the room. What would be most deadly for them in therapy would be to feel invisible or rejected again.

On reviewing an early outline of this project, an esteemed colleague and friend, a writer himself, commented, "It lacks a continuous 'through line' tying it coherently and sequentially together." Upon reflection, I thought, how very fitting! This is precisely the experience of their lives that many of these clients arrive with. Often their knowledge of their histories is spotty, pocked with holes or even blank. I remember a woman once saying, "when I think about my past, I just see bushes; or an occasional image of my dog."

They may not remember anything, or they lack interpersonal memory, as if there was literally no one there. There is no through-line of their lives, and the work of therapy is to create that narrative to thread together the story, and the knowledge that they even have a story. My replicating that lack of "through-line" in my early outline, is an example of how indirect, symbolic and non-verbal communication are often what come to us or through us with these clients. Again, as therapists we must remain keenly aware, including to the clues coming from our own feelings, bodies or inadvertent behavior, that teach us about these clients' world. Since they don't know or have words for much of their experience, often our best information comes to us in other ways, *if* we are listening.

## OVERVIEW OF THE BOOK

### Ancestral Roots

Because so much of what I have learned about neglect is anecdotal and gleaned from my years in the room with many clients, I was inspired to identify the theoretical, conceptual and evidence-based influences that shaped my thinking. Most notably, they are attachment theory; infant neuroscientists such as Allan Schore and the earlier work of Daniel Siegel; and Ruth Lanius' research and integration of ACE data with both mental and physical health and treatment.

### Seeing What Is Not There: Recognizing the "Child of Neglect"

What are the indicators? Chapter 2 lays out some of the immediate clues that the therapist can learn to look for right from the start. Essentially, they all point to the core injury, which for most is the complete and utter failure of mirroring. This, by the way is the missing through-line, in the client's life. Healing from this loss is the fundamental task of the therapy.

## The Therapeutic Relationship: Entering a One-Person World

By definition, the child of neglect is alone too much, and thrown on their own insufficient resources to find the way in the world. The inescapable result is an orientation very much in the first person singular. Most likely, they are unaware of this, or that it is not the norm. Or they may simply be aware that they are less than comfortable in the presence of others; or that they require a lot of "space." The therapeutic relationship is essentially important, complicated and delicate with them. It is definitely not for the faint of heart. A neglect history of one's own is not required, but a depth of empathy most certainly is. Chapter 3 details the requisite skills, qualities and tasks of the therapist for these clients; what kinds of interventions to be aware of, and which also to avoid when possible.

## "But Nothing Happened to Me!" What's the Story?

Because these clients view their histories as being relatively benign or even happy, they may not be open to the idea that something was really missing. Lacking overt trauma such as sexual or physical violence, they may balk or object to the notion. This chapter is designed to help the therapist learn how to discern something of the client's history; and how to begin to speak to them about it, both delicate (and ethically complicated) tasks.

## Emotion: Teaching a Foreign Language

The language of emotion is initially learned by an infant through mirroring. In the absence of that, the world is much more concrete and matter of fact. Emotion may be either a completely alien or unknown entity, or simply irrelevant and void of value. And yet the poverty of emotion does affect them, especially if they are trying to make a go of relationship of some sort. This chapter is designed to help the therapist assess the client's emotional landscape or lack thereof; and how to introduce and access their feelings.

## Sexuality: Unraveling the Conundrum of Need

Although the child of neglect scrupulously finds a way to defy interpersonal need, sex presents a unique challenge. Because although one can indeed conduct a sexual life completely independent of relationship, it is not the same. We must help these clients come to understand and speak about their sexual worlds, and even begin to penetrate or challenge their self-reliance. All of this presents unique challenges, and requires special abilities on the part of the therapist. This chapter begins to navigate that rich world.

## Regulation of Giving: From Resentment to Reciprocity

Because for so many of these people, the primary way they really know how to connect, or be in relationship, is to serve or provide, they may unwittingly fall into "over-giving" or trying unsustainably hard to accommodate; or elaborate unspoken "deals" or assumptions about what they are entitled to or owed as a result. When they ultimately tire or notice what they perceive to be the imbalance, they might become resentful, enraged or even demanding. They may also be oblivious to how rejecting they are of the other's attempts to give to them, or simply experience it as the "wrong thing." Learning to receive is one of the great tasks of the therapy.

## Transforming Shame with Grief with Compassion

Once they understand their own experience, children of neglect acquire acceptance and compassion for the lonely child. This is the goal. They may previously have felt shame about what they lacked, as it has been unintelligible to them or hidden by other preoccupations such as achievement. This is delicate work as they have so painstakingly succeeded at avoidance and denial of emotional vulnerability.

## GPS

This chapter sums up the primary goals and "action items:" for the therapy, which boil down to helping the client to develop "voice" and "spine."

- Teach them to speak aloud: They need to learn how to be visible in relationship rather than disappear, and to speak out loud, rather than withdraw and keep it all inside (which ultimately can result in a smoldering rage). Their previous connections with others have been tenuous and tentative so their default is to "watch and wait," to see if and what the other might do.

- Teach repair skills: I have a protocol I teach called the Lifeboat which is a brief practice they can use to stop an argument by introducing accountability and appreciation rather than blame and criticism. Neglect prevented them from learning the skills of relationship healing and repair, so learning how to reconnect after a rupture is profoundly significant. Repair skills make relationship safe. This discovery makes it safe to make or acknowledge a mistake; and that apology is not failure or defeat.

- Tactfully teach about interpersonal safety: Because self-reliance and feeling independent have become a survival skill for these clients, the idea of repair and interdependence making true intimacy possible may be very threatening, and a formidable challenge. Providing the therapeutic relationship as a laboratory for it, requires great delicacy and skill.

- Reminder of good therapist self-care! Always essential, especially with this challenging population.

## Beyond Words

Other modalities may be useful or essential as talk therapy can be difficult with clients who are not able to verbalize feelings; who feel incapacitated or bored by their lack of a known story; or simply don't know how to access or utilize emotion. Body sensation may be the best way to help them become aware of variations in mood or state. Knowing somatic methodologies is helpful. Referrals for neurofeedback, group therapy, mindfulness-based stress reduction and sometimes support around substance use, may be indicated.

## CONCLUSION

We are hope mongers. In today's world, it is essential to break the intergenerational chain of neglect, which can contribute to violence, poverty, drug addiction and loneliness. It is my fervent desire to help more of us learn how to interrupt this. Sometimes our task is to be the holder of hope when no one else can, to be the one that knows that even though the concert appears to be sold out, we *will* get in. That is the ultimate aim of this book.

## BIBLIOGRAPHY

Amen, Daniel G. *Change Your Brain, Change Your Life: The Breakthrough Program for Conquering Anxiety, Depression, Obsessiveness, Lack of Focus, Anger, and Memory Problems.* Revised ed. New York: Harmony Books, 2015.

Cassidy, Jude, and Phillip R. Shaver, eds. *Handbook of Attachment: Theory, Research, and Clinical Application.* 3rd ed. New York: The Guilford Press, 2016.

Dube, Shanta R., Vincent J. Felitti, Maxia Dong, Daniel P. Chapman, Wayne H. Giles, and Robert F. Anda. "Childhood Abuse, Neglect, and Household Dysfunction and the Risk of Illicit Drug Use: The Adverse Childhood Experiences Study." *Pediatrics* 111, no. 3 (March 2003): 564–572. https://doi.org/10.1542/peds.111.3.564.

Lanius, Ruth A., Eric Vermetten, and Clare Pain, eds. *The Impact of Early Life Trauma on Health and Disease: The Hidden Epidemic.* New York: Cambridge University Press, 2010.

Main, Mary, and Judith Solomon. "Procedures for Identifying Infants as Disorganized/Disoriented During the Ainsworth Strange Situation." In *Attachment in the Preschool Years: Theory, Research, and Intervention*, edited by Mark T. Greenberg, Dante Cicchetti, and E. Mark Cummings, 121–60. Chicago: University of Chicago Press, 1990.

McGilchrist, Iain. *The Master and His Emissary: The Divided Brain and the Making of the Western World.* Expanded ed. New Haven: Yale University Press, 2009.

Ogden, Thomas H. *Projective Identification and Psychotherapeutic Technique.* New York: Routledge, 2018. First published 1982 by Jason Aronson (New York).

Schore, Allan N. *Affect Regulation and the Origin of the Self: The Neurobiology of Emotional Development.* New York: Routledge, 2016. First published 1994 by Lawrence Erlbaum Associates (Hillsdale, New Jersey).

Shapiro, Francine, and Margot Silk Forrest. *EMDR: The Breakthrough Therapy for Overcoming Anxiety, Stress, and Trauma.* New York: Basic Books, 2016.

Siegel, Daniel J. *The Developing Mind: How Relationships and the Brain Interact to Shape Who We Are.* 3rd ed. New York: The Guilford Press, 2020.

Van der Kolk, Bessel A. "Developmental Trauma Disorder: A New, Rational Diagnosis for Children with Complex Trauma Histories." *Psychiatric Annals* 35, no. 5 (May 2005): 401–408.

Van der Kolk, Bessel A., Alexander C. McFarlane, and Lars Weisaeth, eds. *Traumatic Stress: The Effects of Overwhelming Experience on Mind, Body, and Society.* New York: The Guilford Press, 1996.

# Chapter 2

# Seeing What Isn't There: Recognizing the "Child of Neglect"

To reconstruct, or construct for the first time a coherent autobiographical narrative, out of fractured and fragmented bits and pieces of memory, is a core task of all trauma work. It is difficult and painstaking, invariably slow. That will be our objective when we get to it. The first task for the therapist, however, is to recognize the child of neglect, to identify that neglect is what we are dealing with. To begin with, most survivors of neglect do not know they have a story. They may arrive with an elaborate story about someone else. Especially because I am a relationship therapist, this is often what I see. They may present with a partner, who may have corralled them into coming; with a passionate desire to get their partner "fixed;" or for a post mortem about a confusingly failed relationship. And there are those who just don't understand why they feel lousy or empty, or depressed. The first order of business is assessment, for *us* as therapists to discern not only why they think they are there, but also why *we* think they are there. This is decidedly delicate work. Of course, we want to be scrupulously respectful, and never have the hubris or professional grandiosity to imply that we know better than they do about them! And as we will see later, with neglect comes a particular sensitivity about knowing what they know, about themselves and everything else really. So the therapist must roll up their sleeves and take their time, which may collide with what is often the client's impatience to get on with it.

I am a veteran of the "false memory syndrome" nightmare of the 1990s when at a mass level, trauma survivors and their therapists were accused of fabricating and implanting memories of abuse out of "imagination" and "fantasy;" charging parents with "allegations" of maltreatment and crimes. It created havoc in families; terrorized therapists who worked with trauma; and confused the public about the function of memory, and specifically traumatic memory which was just coming to be understood. The trauma field as a whole, and its practitioners, not to mention the already suffering clients took a walloping hit.

I want to be very cautious here. We do *not* want to make up a childhood for our neglect (or any) clients or have them invent a painful fiction for themselves. In the case of neglect, however, they are highly unlikely to do that, as their tendency is much more in the direction of minimizing or denying. In fact, that may in itself be a flag, or a hint to take note of.

Similarly, we are *not* out to villainize often traumatized, impoverished or well-meaning parents. We simply want to accurately identify these survivors of neglect so they themselves, can understand what is "wrong." Most of what I have come to refer to as the "Neglect Profile" I have gleaned from observation over three plus decades, correlating it to theory and brain science where possible, updating my files as I and we as a field learned and continue to learn more.

## ANOTHER DILEMMA WITHOUT SOLUTION

When Jackie (Not her real name of course, and all identifying information has been changed to protect her confidentiality, as with all case examples throughout this book;) first came to me, she had been in therapy for 15 years with a therapist she liked well enough. Although it had always been "nice," to have someone to talk to, she felt she was not making progress, and wondered if something or someone else might be more helpful. Of course, I wanted to know what she meant by "progress." I found that was not so simple to get to.

Jackie had a lifelong eating disorder. Beginning as far back as she could remember, her mother always took her to the "chubby" department, and from the time she started school, she was always the "fat girl." In those days, she remarked, there were usually only one or two in each grade. By the time she was nine, Jackie's mother was delivering her at least weekly, to Weight Watchers, which was an agony for her, and which she was never "successful" at. Jackie always felt like an outcast, and for all of her school years, she suffered from loneliness. She could only conclude, that her weight was the reason she could not make friends. Her mother's only noticeable intervention was depositing her at Weight Watchers; and for a while at swim team. But for the most part, her mother had her nose in a book. Jackie's sadness and her ballooning young waistline, went largely ignored. Food continued to be her only reliable companion, both the source of comfort and the source of threat, Jackie's dilemma without solution. It became her secret world of shame and solace, and continued to be throughout her life. Food continued to be the primary relationship, and so there was no other.

A bright woman, Jackie did well in school and went to college and graduate school, and became a well-loved helping professional. Caretaking became her social world, and work and the food obsession, her preoccupations. Living again in her hometown, Jackie's main recreational companion became her aging mother, who was rarely too busy to share a sporting event, a movie, or a meal out. Although her relationship with her mom was vapid and disconnected, it was "nice" to have someone to do things with.

Two years prior to our meeting, Jackie had had an expensive, painful and medically elaborate gastric bypass surgery. She got her hopes way up that this would change her life. At first it did with dramatic medical complications, that landed her first in the emergency room and then in the hospital for several weeks. But she had lost 145 pounds from the surgery. What came next, to Jackie's horror and devastating disappointment, was that she soon gained back most of it. What was most troubling to her, however, was that despite her continued individual therapy, and a post-surgery therapy group facilitated by her "weight doctor," *no one seemed to see* what was happening as the weight crept back, inquire, or help her get a handle on it. She felt alone, invisible, powerless, and hopelessly depressed, all feelings that were painfully familiar.

Jackie was bright and likeable, yet our early sessions had a "sleepy" quality to them. She made virtually no eye contact, and it was difficult to feel connected. I often felt she was not quite with me in the room. And although she identified the "weight issue." And her "obsession" with it, as the problem that brought her, she rarely if ever spoke explicitly about it. At this point, I can barely remember what we did talk about.

One redundant dynamic between us did become lively in those early days. It was illustrative, as was my repeatedly falling back in the same hole. Clearly, Jackie was trying to teach me something. Although Jackie was quite private about her actual eating patterns and habits, she would vociferously and deeply despair about *not knowing what to do.* I would unwittingly slip into problem-solving mode, asking questions that infuriated her and made me one more person who did not get it, or who insulted her with ideas of things to "try" that she had exhausted over a lifetime of suffering about weight. She hated going to any kind of medical appointment, not only because she despised being directed to step on the odious scale, but more because they all invariably insulted her with the instruction to "eat less and exercise more." If she could do that, would there be a multi-zillion dollar weight loss industry? And did they really think she did not know it? Any idiot knew that! The last thing she wanted from me was ideas of what to "do." How many times would I misunderstand her despair as a cry for "practical" help?

To Jackie, exercise was an agony and a punishing penance. Any mention of it enraged her. What she needed, and did not know she needed, was an accurate mirror, not of her body. She needed her pain and desperate frustration to be seen, and she needed help finding the language for the unrelenting and unbearable emotions, that perpetuated the complex behavior, which also served as a numbing device. She did not know what it was she was crying out for, but she clearly knew what it wasn't. And no one else had ever seen or "gotten it;" not her "rail thin" therapist of 15 years, not the weight loss doctor or her group members, not her med psychiatrist, and certainly not her mother. When I finally caught wind of what I was doing, paid enough attention to *her* to actually observe and think about my own behavior and its impact; named it, owned it and stopped it, something dramatically opened between us.

It is hard to describe the change, but gradually Jackie came into focus. As I awoke to presence with her, she appeared to do the same. We began to make authentic contact, and the emphasis was no longer on weight. She did begin to talk some about what she was eating, but it was more than anything symbolic, a way of saying "you are not like the others, I can tell you." But the subject did not hold her interest anymore. She began to realize for herself, slowly, that food was not really the point.

## THE FAILURE OF MIRRORING

The primary missing experience of neglect is the failure of mirroring. From the earliest ages, Jackie felt that no one saw she was there, or reflected what they saw. Jackie's mother was a bookworm, and although she did not work outside the home, Jackie really did not know what her mother did all day, except that she saw the growing piles of books around the house. And she dutifully had dinner on the table promptly at 5:00 each day, when Jackie's irritable and demanding father came home.

Dinner was never pleasant. Her parents did not get along well. There was little conversation. Jackie's mother was not a bad cook, but there was no pleasure to be had in meal times together. And no one spoke to her. It was easy for a little girl to wonder why she was invisible. Did she even exist? Was she worthy of existence? Or did she simply not matter? These questions were not consciously known to her or clearly cognitively formulated for a long time. Rather they resided in emotion, or expressed themselves in attitudes, body experience and behavior.

Sometimes Jackie's mother forgot to pick her up from swim practice, and the little girl stood shivering on a street corner as darkness descended, long before we had cell phones. She never noticed, asked or listened to Jackie's distress and perennial failure with the dreaded Weight Watchers. It did not seem to command her attention that Jackie had no friends, perhaps because she didn't either. Jackie and her sister, circulated like ghosts in the house, not interacting much even with each other. Jackie's mother remained blithely unaware that the child was perennially downcast.

Jackie's absence of eye contact grabbed my attention, as noted. As a culture, we have long viewed the eyes as the "windows on the soul," and this is true in many cultures. We now have hard data and neuroimaging scans that corroborate the fear associated with direct eye contact in those with histories of some sort of trauma, as compared with those who do not. An infant child, (or anyone really) looks into the eyes of another, to assess danger or safety. It is the primitive fear center that is activated to take a reading. If there is a calm and apparently favorable response in the eyes of the other, the social engagement and more highly evolved brain areas are activated, and even a release of oxytocin, pleasure and ease. Ruth Lanius' lab carefully studied this. In research subjects who had experienced trauma or neglect, the brain stayed in the alarm state and did not advance to the higher cortical social engagement area. The sense of danger and threat installed the impulse to avoid, which became the default. So, absence of eye contact can be one of our markers or flags of a neglect history, as well as being a presentation of shame. As Schore makes clear, the infant brain develops in resonance with the mother's brain, right hemisphere to right hemisphere, through the gaze. It becomes easy to wonder about a deficit of gazing. It was certainly easy to wonder that about Jackie.

Because it is highly unusual for me to feel bored in a client session, I have learned to notice, rather than reprimand myself. An infant left alone too much will be lonely, scared, not to mention hungry, possibly wet and cold, interminably "waiting," and most likely lifelessly bored. So boredom and waiting being exaggeratedly dreaded, is another marker I have come to recognize as possibly pointing to a neglect history. Boredom is experienced as deathly. My client Hank would routinely incite wildly provocative and volatile political arguments when a dinner party or family holiday felt lifeless, to interrupt the unbearable boredom.

When I am feeling inordinately tired, stealing too many glances at the clock, or overly enthusiastic anticipating my dinner, there is a clue. I have come to know that my experience of myself is my richest resource with these clients. My brilliant neurofeedback consultant repeatedly reminds me, "Whenever a neurofeedback client, (or I myself,) experiences any thought, feeling or behavior that is out of the ordinary, we never rule out the possibility that neurofeedback is a factor." I would say the same here: Any atypical experience of myself may very well be a communication about the inner world of the client, that they are unable to express to me, or that I have failed to "hear." (Of course, it may also be my personal neurofeedback! I must have the self-awareness to assess that too.)

I think of my client, Howard, with whom I was exploring a devastating romantic relationship break-up. He had been struggling for several years to get over it. My general reaction to Robin, his ex, was to feel protective of him, a sorely missing experience from his abandonment ridden childhood, and an anger and annoyance with Robin. I was careful not to appear overly critical of her. And to manage any judgment I felt. He seemed to appreciate the empathy, and what also seemed to accurately reflect his bitterness about her dismissiveness, insensitivity, and what seemed to him wanton rejections of him. Our work and our collaboration seemed to me to be going well.

One evening I was driving home from work, and heard a story on the radio, about a local humanitarian organization that I had never heard of before. I found myself thinking, "Wow, that would be a good place for Robin to work." I knew that she had been rather a lost soul professionally, and searching for meaningful work, and meaning in general. Suddenly I felt great compassion for Robin and sympathy for how lost she felt. I had never felt any such sad and open-hearted feelings about Robin in all the months I had been working with Howard. That struck me. In our next session, I inquired about how we were doing with processing the relationship. Howard admitted, not without shame, that he had spent two days crying about Robin, and actually missed a day of work, feeling immobilized by his grief. My unusual thought was informing me of what I was failing to perceive, and Howard was unable to tell me. His eagerness to put it all behind him once and for all, neglected the well of emotion I was missing. Had I not noticed my own aberrant thought and feeling, I would have continued to miss his.

Therapist self-reflection and mindfulness are a crucially necessary part of the data collection, and are to be not necessarily assumed, but considered. One of the innumerable costs of the Pandemic that we must work extra hard to mitigate, is how working remotely decidedly dulls and mutes the many subtle and not-so-subtle sensory cues of a live exchange.

With Jackie, a first hint was when I felt the weight of sleepiness. Then finding that the lack of eye contact annoyed me, also uncharacteristic for me. Registering those experiences, I attempted, to quietly translate what Jackie herself could not verbalize. What might she be needing to communicate to me about her experience of being unseen? It was more than pain and fear. It was also bitter frustration and anger and confusion. After all she had not asked to be born. Why would they bother to bring her into the world, only to then "disappear" her into non-existence? Of course, it was a long time before I could point it out or inquire about it.

Anger, was not a state Jackie could recognize or own, certainly in childhood it was way too dangerous. "Anger was a luxury, something that only skinny, pretty girls could afford to have, let alone express. They would still be liked. I already had to work overtime to try and get people to like me. And already nobody did. I didn't dare give them more reasons to reject me?" And it was perhaps forbidden, or a domain only permissible to her chronically grumpily aggressive father, which admittedly and guiltily made her not like him too much. Also, much later in our work we identified, that Jackie was infinitely more inclined to experience anger as agitated hunger, something to be assuaged with ice cream, or her other most loved foods which were hard and crunchy.

No speculation is required to understand the grief and pain of not being "worthy of notice." Paul Ekman, a world expert on emotion, has identified the universal facial expressions of the full range of human emotions. He found averted eyes and avoidance of eye contact to be international expressions of shame. With Jackie, it did fit. She was always somewhat hiding, Granted, she was always baffled by the irony, that fat people are so conspicuous and simultaneously so invisible. But she was more comfortable with hiddenness, and most certainly kept her eating urgently concealed. The weight served as a barrier to hide behind. In her work as a helping professional, she was exquisitely effective and efficient. She could hide in her role, and not ever be truly known, even feeling some satisfaction while doing it. People responded favorably, even appreciatively to Jackie the helper, so she could take pleasure in that without risking the rejection she was sure she would feel if she were truly known.

Rejection is a default mode for these clients. They will sniff it out and interpret it anywhere, including in the therapist. In couples work, I have not infrequently been accused of favoring the other partner, or in an extreme case, even trying to steal him from the painfully neglected woman. So even with the utmost of caution, we also can be viewed through that critical, rejecting lens. If there are cases where it may in fact be true, if we truly do not like the person, we must work all the harder to be equidistant, or if necessary, refer out. Rejection is a ready explanation for neglect. "I am un-interesting, undesirable, ugly, stupid;" in Jackie's case, "fat." That is the ready "rationale" for the inattention. "I have no reason to exist, no right to occupy space in this world." Nothing else seems to make sense.

Existence weaves in and out as a theme, and the conundrum of existence shows itself all kinds of ways. I early on noticed a tendency with many of these clients, that at first, I experienced as a kind of contrariness, that could even feel at times like argumentativeness. I learned It is not angry, but adamant, a kind of reflexive seemingly urgent and rapid-fire push-back. It was as if agreeing with me might be on the order of annihilation. I might summarize back virtually verbatim, what they had just said, and when I inquire if I had understood accurately, invariably I might hear "no." And get a correction, that to me, sounded precisely like what I had just said. This is not to say I never make a mistake, of course, I do. But the pattern is to perennially disagree, differ or *distinguish* me from you, as if existence would require that "I am clearly *not* you, but someone *distinct*. And perhaps if I am not *you, I* might have a shot at being seen." Of course, this becomes a point of conflict in couples, where a partner may tire of what feels like a chronic "argument" or correction, or one-upping. And admittedly it can be exhausting for us.

My repeated "argument" with Jackie, however, was a different one. Since no one had ever taught her either to identify or to express emotion, her asking for help with that, could sound very much like a request to problem-solve together. When she lamented and despaired about what to do, she did not want to hear inquiries or suggestions about exercise and self-regulation, or treatment approaches. She repeatedly told me what she wanted because I in fact did not get it. It would have been preferable for me to self-reflect enough to figure that out myself, so she wouldn't have to keep trying to tell me. On the day I finally said, "Problem solving is something you have always found ways to do, even before we had google and Wikipedia, with your resourceful, ferocious, self-reliance. I am not going to step in that hole again!" she looked up and smiled, heaving a long and breathy sigh. She did not have words, but the language of her body was her way of saying "Thank you! At last!" She even met my eyes and stayed there for a nanosecond. Perhaps, just maybe in this relationship, she did not have to do it all. Well just maybe.

## FLAGS AND MARKERS

In our culture of "Rugged Individualism," certainly in the United States, the fact that we are pack animals, designed and built for interdependence, may be a hard sell. For the child of neglect, where self-reliance is not a choice but an only option, a survival mechanism and a defense against the despair of loneliness and abandonment, it may also be a point of pride. So, finding a "role" with these clients can be a challenge. They often do not realize how rejecting they themselves might seem, so accustomed to being the rejected one. Often, they themselves are mystified as to why they are in my office.

Thomas, who came for couple's therapy with his spouse of several decades, was a case in point. He was desperately miserable, wanted to shout from the rooftops how much pain he was in. For the life of me, I could not figure it out for quite a while. I liked him. He was bright, and even, when not on a rant, funny. He was powerfully successful in the world, and proud of it. He made a good life for his family, and his wife had stayed home to raise their now teenage kids, whom he unabashedly adored. I could not figure out how he felt about her either. But his anger went zero to 100 at the speed of light, so I had to be quick on my feet to keep the temperature between them such that we could work.

Thomas characterized his family of origin as perfect and ideal, and it was besides being an unbearable agony, a point of shame to find himself in marital discord, and God forbid, therapy. It was a secret from his family and definitely from their kids. And Thomas was decidedly annoyed with me for not being helpful and repeatedly returned to the refrain of "what the hell are we doing here?" Needless to say, the evenings after their sessions required extra self-care for me, and also special attention to the indirect ways I might be getting information. He also canceled our sessions fairly often due to his very important job. If I ever dared to point out that or spotty schedule did not facilitate progress, he would just be incensed, and feel unheard. I rapidly learned to cut that out.

Thomas, to his wife's chagrin, had no interest in looking at his childhood. She was a bright, and avid reader of self-help books, and considered herself the epitome of emotional-intelligence. Her authoritative responses to him were lightning quick and had a superior sounding tone of impatience. Thomas rarely had a moment to even see for himself that he was not quite able to recognize, let alone express, what he was feeling. Searching for how I could help, I considered, perhaps my primary function for Thomas was to clear the space and make the *time* for him to formulate and learn the words to express himself, which points to another marker.

Another note-worthy flag of neglect is the *pace* at which the individual might communicate and process. This may be most evident in a couple, but certainly not exclusively. Thomas expressed himself with long pauses. The days when he had nothing in mind to talk about, and "nothing to say" were the ones where he contacted the greatest depth, when we cleared the space. Often, I functioned as an insistent snow-plow, clearing a path where the car can roll. Where Thomas's wife's reaction was usually to flame quickly to anger or impatience that he had nothing to say, given the opportunity he had a lot to say. That was when we learned about how deeply rejected and lonely, he felt. (Of course, Thomas's wife also had a story, and in couple's work, we must attend to both sides. In the service of our focus on neglect, we are purposely not examining her side of the equation here.)

Assuming a failure of right hemisphere to right hemisphere gazing, (in Thomas's case purely a hypothesis since he had so little to say about his childhood,) we can surmise that the right hemisphere, which is the locus of more emotion and subjectivity, would be understimulated, and therefore slower. Nonetheless, when I quietly assumed my snow-plow function, at least I felt like I was offering *something*, especially if I didn't call attention to it. Thomas resolutely insisted the therapy wasn't helping, that he did not feel less miserable or desperate in his marriage, but every time I intervened to slow down his wife, and attempted to subtly teach the vocabulary of emotion, he appeared immensely comforted, relieved and calmed, and felt much more confident to speak with her.

To teach the vocabulary of emotion, I might offer a menu of feeling words: "Do you mean, hurt? sad; frustrated? mad? resigned?" Usually he would reject them all, but given the time, he would find his own words. The magic was in the time, largely waiting, and enduring sometimes very long silences, which might evoke a memory, even a song. It became unmistakable to me what my function was, or what Thomas might "need" me for. And of course, I knew not to say it. Sometimes an acknowledgment of progress, might even come across as patting myself on the back, or might hit the gnarly terrain of receiving, which we will explore later.

For those who are less responsive to the menu of words, an access route may be to ask, "What are you aware of feeling in your body?" Although strangers to emotion they may have more fluency at locating body sensations, which can lead us to emotion. Some clients may have no interest at all in that question, or find it even more annoying. They may be lifelong sufferers from somatic or body related complaints that may be another expression of the story, as in the case of Jackie for one, and profoundly disconnected, dis-identified from, or antagonistic toward their bodies. But there are those for whom it is a powerful way of teaching about the integration body and emotion in a way that makes for a heightened sense of wholeness.

Self-reliance is the necessary default when there is no one there. It is necessary to survival. Needing a therapist may be an affront to that, an insult, a narcissistic injury or a threat. Attempting to answer Thomas's question "why am I here?" would be like problem solving with Jackie about her weight. It is hearing the wrong question. We must go gently and quietly around self-reliance. Either they will come to discover their need and connect with us as Jackie did, or they will eventually (from my standpoint prematurely) leave, as Thomas ultimately did.

Self-reliance, "help resistance" or rejection of the therapist role, (let alone the actual therapist) is a marker to be duly noted. Clients may at times, like Thomas, experience themselves frustrated or even desperate in their efforts for what they experience as their "needs" to be comprehended. And they may simply just not see how difficult that might be for another to grasp. They don't see how incomplete their communication might be, especially if they are as bright as Thomas.

Another ready clue to a neglect history, is the ready default to "I don't know" as the perennial answer to the question of what they are feeling or what they want, even what they might like. They may insist that they have no idea, and appear to collapse into a helpless shame ridden passivity. Of course, this again reflects the failure of mirroring, and the poverty of time and interest anyone might have had to listen, or to help them learn how to speak. And how do we help them to know what they know? I might say (and humor is an essential ingredient in this difficult work!) "You don't get to stop at 'I don't know'" or "You don't get to say that here." Then I wait. With sufficient time, like Thomas, they may be eloquent, even surprised by tears.

The same was true for Elisa, who was the youngest of nine children, and grew up in a family of impassioned and frantically busy political activists. What she also most needed, and similarly what was perhaps all she could take in for this run of therapy, was the time; an interested, attentive other; and some "emotional education." Elisa was a child of the 1960s when the world was aflame with so many causes: the Vietnam War; Black Power, Civil Rights, Labor Unions, to name a few. Everyone was so busy and serious, and it all seemed so important. Elisa had no idea what was going on. So many grown-ups that she did not know trooped in and out of their small apartment in the projects, and it seemed as if there were secrets, things to not tell anyone outside the family. But Elisa had no idea what they were, or what all this very important commotion was about. No one took the time to explain it, or address her confusion and fear. I always had the image of a little girl being virtually stomped underfoot by the loud rhythmic pounding of combat boots echoing in their over-crowded home. She vanished in the dizzying uproar, feeling invisible, insignificant, or in the way.

Elisa grew up lonely and feeling chronically empty, and guilty for not making a dramatic political commitment. To be honest, she really did not care that much about politics, but she could not possibly admit that. She came into therapy still not quite knowing what was going on, now inside of her, and now close to 50. She had chosen a partner who was also very busy and important. The relationship awakened feelings that seemed oddly familiar but she could not quite place them.

Elisa knew that she was drinking too much. She was tired of feeling lonely. But again, did not know why she had come to therapy. Just slowing time, to help her even tune in to her inner experience, and an interested, present other was a new experience for her. It stunned her how dazzled she felt just to have someone remember what she had said last week. As she recognized how invisible and forgotten, how worthless and alone she had always felt, there was a flood of grief that went on for quite a time. But there was also great relief in finding an explanation for how she had always felt. The idea that perhaps it was not true that she was uninteresting or worthless; could it be possible that it was not all her "fault?" That too was a huge relief and motivated her to be visible.

Elisa was a small business owner, a mother, and had created an elaborately sustainable home and garden. She even kept bees, which I was most impressed by. Becoming visible to herself was a start, and she noticed that she did feel better. It was still difficult to regulate her drinking. She did not stay in therapy too long. That also sometimes happens. Opening the well of need, may be more of a life change than the client can bear. I am not sure if the drinking got the better of Elisa. Often, they come back, sometimes years later. Sometimes not.

Another marker may be the idyllic, perfect scenario of childhood. Sallie grew up on a flower farm. What could be more picturesque than that? She might describe the irresistibly blooming fields, especially to a nature lover like me. It might be easy to miss how many chores that Sallie had to complete before running for the school bus. As early as kindergarten, she knew no category for feeling, because there was neither time nor the option of diverging from the unending requirements of caring for growing things (other than herself of course!) She was proud to be so handy and so resourceful, and she loved animals and plants. She painted and thought of the scenery of her childhood as charming and rather quaint; her salt of the earth parents as decent and hearty folk who did the best they could. In these times, it is not easy to make it as a small farmer in a world of industrialized agriculture. Even though she did not want that life for herself now, she could see how hard her parents had always worked. Sallie appreciated that. She really did not want to find any fault with them or her upbringing. But she was interested in understanding better why she was so fiercely autonomous and untrusting of others. A note of caution, the therapist must be mindful, and not swept by a romantic or poetic impressionistic painting of a childhood, that may obstruct the view of what the client needs for us to see. Perhaps that is also all that the world has ever seen of them.

In some cases, having the space cleared for the child of neglect to find their feeling is welcome. It may alternatively or additionally bring fear or overwhelm. As my inordinately rational and unemotional mother said of her Holocaust experience, "We were afraid if we started to cry, we would never stop." I later learned that James Baldwin had said something very similar. So, keeping it buttoned up tight was protection. And time and attention for feeling may also bring contempt, as living without emotion for as long as they have, may have been adaptive, and even a way to feel superior.

Self-reliance points to the missing experience of having someone to turn to, someone to think of as a resource, a protector, mentor or container for the pain, fear, and the many challenges of inner and outer life. The child of neglect, does not "know" that interpersonal need is both natural and inevitable, that we are born a bundle of needs, and that we are among the last to emerge from dependency on parents, of the mammal world. Because it is at best inconvenient, and at worst life threatening, the child of neglect defaults to a disavowal of interpersonal need. Or they try.

During the Pandemic, Alex was unnerved by how the "lockdown" thrust him "prematurely" into interdependence with a relatively new partner. "Because Robert was the only person with whom I had direct, face to face contact over these months, I had to get used to having one 'go to' person for even company." But having been in therapy for some time, and recognizing that he was working through his neglect, he rather appreciated the way circumstances gave him a push.

Although there will be much more to say about self-reliance later, one interesting koan or paradox is worth presenting here. Alongside the conscious or unconscious and often ferocious self-reliance, resides a profound powerlessness or helplessness in the interpersonal. Thomas's wife would leap into a boiling rage when on a rough day between them, Thomas would say to her plaintively, "I'll just sit here and wait until the sun comes out," essentially declaring he would passively sit there until *she* would "snap out of it," making it all OK for both of them. He truly believed it was all up to her.

This is another hallmark: "There is nothing I can do," in the interpersonal. A similarly familiar refrain is "I don't know what to do!" We begin to get the picture of a desolation about which they had virtually no impact. If they cried or acted out, excelled or failed, or like Jackie, gained life-threatening amounts of weight, chances were slim that they would garner a flicker of attention by their efforts. Or if they did get that smidgen, they did not know why. Attention or no attention seemed completely arbitrary in the eyes of the lonely child, and completely outside their control. Thomas's wife found this lament blaming, unflattering and often insulting. The child of neglect can be both fiercely self-reliant and utterly powerless.

Similarly, we find among these clients another paradox, about knowing. The child of neglect often presents as a "know it all" which may have the unwanted consequence that people in fact don't like them. Most likely there was no one to ask about most things, so they had to find their own answers. And survival may have depended on that. They may also have made themselves "expert" at analyzing and knowing how others felt and what the other may be thinking, even if their expertise or conclusions were skewed.

Searching for something to orient to, they find or create their own explanations, and may become adamantly attached to them. Because their own analyses may have served them like life rafts when they were adrift in childhood, or as a buffer against facing the terror of not knowing, they operate by a unique belief system. The distortion is most glaring and most useful (if challenging) if it is about me.

Bill, a therapist was convinced I was in competition with him and out to steal his ideas and his clients. I later learned that he had had a brother just like that. Horribly neglected by their mother, he had to guard against the meager crumbs of attention he might occasionally get, being quickly scooped up by this brother, who simultaneously postured to out-do and outshine him to get more; while also bullying him brutally. Seeing the contrast between what he believed I thought and felt, and what I actually did think and feel was both shocking and illuminating. Again, one of the rich ways of learning the story together, if a more difficult part of our job!

So, as they desperately "don't know" what to do interpersonally, the child of neglect simultaneously knows everything about the other; and often collapses into the despair of immobility and hopeless helplessness. They may also in the midst of having all the answers about the world, walk around completely bereft in not knowing "Am I doing enough?" "Am I doing OK?" "Am I doing the right things?" "what should I do?" and in effect, dizzy and tortured by the unrelenting *not* knowing.

## SUMMING UP AND WHAT TO DO

What we are attempting to do in this chapter, is learn to recognize when neglect is an essential issue, and what some of the markers are for a working hypothesis. I emphasize, that we must utilize and rely on much more than the client's telling us directly and verbally, because they may have very incomplete knowledge themselves. This is not a "cookie cutter" process, and we certainly do not want to hastily apply the neglect lens. The therapist's whole body, imagination, emotional spectrum, and intellect will be required, which means our own subjectivity and biases must also be kept in view. And in.

turn, we must not become overly attached (or obviously so!) to our own subjectivity. That being said some of the markers and data points I have collected over the years include:

- Noticing uncharacteristic feelings or behaviors in myself. This may include boredom, sleepiness, feeling the weight of time, and being perhaps distracted or distractable, which is for me out of the ordinary. Of course, each and every therapist has their own set of vulnerabilities, and their own repertoire of what may be characteristic and usual, so self-awareness is as ever, crucial.

- Other markers include a desperate cry of "I don't know what to do!" or "There is nothing I can do." This may seem strangely in contrast to how competent they might appear in the world. It may point to an interpersonal world where they had no impact, and sought hopelessly to find a way to win or attract attention and care.

- Ironically and simultaneously "knowing it all," having been thrown on their own resources to figure out how the world works, and being often fiercely attached and defensive, about what they "know."

- A kind of contrariness or argumentativeness.

- Disavowal of interpersonal need. It was both disastrously unsafe, and painfully pointless to need anything from another. Creating a fortress of independence, and a myth of self-sufficiency is a mode of survival. It is more than a belief-system, it is a necessity. It also may be so familiar, that like ambient air, it is outside of awareness. But the therapist may notice a certain distance that the client appears to keep, and perhaps an acute ambivalence about therapy.

- Sparse memory of childhood, particularly in the interpersonal. This adds up to a vague or missing narrative or autobiographical story, and of course, makes it harder to dis-spell myths and idealization about a perfectly fine and uneventful background.

- An absence of eye contact.

- Vulnerability and acute sensitivity to criticism and rejection. Criticism being rapidly interpreted as rejection.

- Questions about existence, including, what constitutes worthiness to exist.
- Emotional flatness, or a foreignness to emotion or even its relevance.

Most of this process of observation and data collection go on quietly inside the therapist, while we are occupied with the generic task of getting to know the client and creating safety. Later comes the task of bringing into focus or piecing together a largely unknown, spotty, fractured or "romanticized" story, and similarly what is "needed" for healing. With creative use of all the senses; a good and compassionate consultant, plenty of humility, patience, willingness to troubleshoot and learn from mistakes; and willingness to take the *time*, we like Michelangelo, will unveil the sculpture hidden inside the stone.

## BIBLIOGRAPHY

Baldwin, James. *No Name in the Street.* New York: Dial Press, 1972.

Ekman, Paul. *Emotions Revealed: Recognizing Faces and Feelings to Improve Communication and Emotional Life.* Revised ed. New York: Owl Books, 2003.

Pope, Kenneth. "Memory, Abuse, and Science: Questioning Claims about the False Memory Syndrome Epidemic." *American Psychologist* 51, no. 9 (September 1996): 957–974. https://doi.org/10.1037/0003-066X.51.9.957.

Schore, Allan N. *Affect Regulation and the Origin of the Self: The Neurobiology of Emotional Development.* New York: Routledge, 2016. First published 1994 by Lawrence Erlbaum Associates (Hillsdale, New Jersey).

Steuwe, Carolin, Judith K. Daniels, Paul A. Frewen, Maria Densmore, Sebastian Pannasch, Thomas Beblo, Jeffrey Reiss, and Ruth A Lanius. "Effect of Direct Eye Contact in PTSD Related to Interpersonal Trauma: An fMRI Study of Activation of an Innate Alarm System." *Social Cognitive and Affective Neuroscience* 9, no. 1 (January 2014): 88–97. https://doi.org/10.1093/scan/nss105.

# Chapter 3

# The Therapeutic Relationship: Entering a One Person World

Examining the therapeutic relationship is a visit to the interpersonal world of these clients. Perhaps this is true of all our clients. However, with the adult child of neglect, it feels somehow more glaring or more fraught. For the most part, their experience with a caregiver was primarily absence or blankness at best, so they may not have a category for why relationship would be important. And a relationship with a paid stranger? That often makes no sense at all.

I remember when I began therapy at age 28, my therapist was a cloud of fog in the corner of the room, which seemed miles away from me. It took me several years before I saw the outlines of a human being in a chair. It is hard to fathom what it was like to sit with me! I had to come for sessions multiple times per week, because I could not imagine I would be remembered from one day to the literal next. If she let me, I would have constantly given my therapist things for her office, some artifact or reminder that I existed. It was my experience to be "out of sight, out of mind," or in my world, out of existence. It was a long road for us.

The work with neglect, begins an ironic challenge. On one hand, what these clients need most urgently, what they most respond to, thrive and grow from in the therapy, is this relationship. Yet on the other, that is the last thing that they think they need, and certainly the last thing they would want. Like Jackie, they may think the "issue" is something else, or Howard, wanting to understand what went wrong in what seemed like the love of his life.

Often, they are confused or don't understand what might make the therapy relationship important. "Why do you want to talk about that?" Or "why do you keep calling attention to yourself?" For example, the question, "what are you feeling about my upcoming two-week vacation?" They might view such a question as a show of narcissism, self-aggrandizement or a self-importance on my part, which may have echoes in their past. It may seem like a waste of their time and money, or as if I am asking them to take care of me. Howard was usually only aware of my absence as being a break from the gnawing expense. Jim might look forward to having his schedule free of interruptions. "I won't have to get out of bed if I don't want to." And the child of neglect may even be ambivalent about the ordeal of relationship in general. Only sometime later, could Jackie see how dysregulating it was for her when I was not there. Needless to say, at least at first, it is a tightrope to walk, but a highly informative one nonetheless. The therapeutic relationship is our first and best window into what the experiences of their caregivers was like. Nothing particularly unique about that, except for the salience of it, and the fact that we may not get a lot of other information. What I will generally say to the client at this stage, is "Please, if ever I say or do something that misses the mark, or God forbid, hurts your feelings, please tell me! It is very important that I not do that to you." And sometimes I am very surprised even enlightened by what I learn.

For example, Carolyn, a child of neglect, I saw now many years ago, was an avid social justice activist. This was long before public awareness of implicit bias and unconscious racism was anything like what it is today. However, racial equality and justice had always been very important to me. I had only known this beautiful African-American woman with elaborate hair weaves, multiple braids or dreadlocks. One day she showed up with scrupulously processed arrow straight hair.

As a Jewish girl growing up in the 60s, I viewed my exceptionally curly hair as a curse, and always jealously coveted straight hair, preferably long straight hair. When Carolyn showed up with long, "perfectly" straight hair I immediately complimented her, perhaps even effusively. I noticed a subtle but undeniably chilly change between after that. Only when I inquired if something had happened between us, did I learn that she was participating in a study, measuring how differently African Americans were seen or treated in the world when they looked more "white." Affronted by my racism exposed, she felt hideously unseen and unappreciated for who she was. I was "exposed" as another pseudo-progressive fake, and not to be trusted. It was my first glimpse at Carolyn's mother, who was not only neglectful, self-important and abandoning, but also deceitful in how she presented herself in the world. Carolyn may have left therapy had we not explored this change, and gone deeper than the obvious, that I was just one more racist white lady.

A childhood of neglect was most often a vast open empty expanse of solitude. The client may or may not even be aware of it, or aware that this is out of the ordinary, or not the natural order. It is their ambient air. Additionally, if they have experienced more overt trauma and/or violence, they might think of *that* as the primary problem.

Lisa's sexual abuse perpetrators were numerous. Because sex and relationships with men were so problematic in her life, she viewed the sexual abuse and those men, as the source of her trauma symptoms. And indeed, to some extent they were. However, even though her mother's eruptions of rage and violence, and overt and severe physical abuse against her, were not infrequent, she continued to see the men as having done the harm. Admittedly I was horrified to hear the stories about some of the beatings at her mother's hands (and other chilling implements!) She could not see how her mother's neglect could hold a candle to sexual abuse, even though it began probably at birth. It did not seem to dawn on her that neglect can enable failures of protection or detection to occur. And early neglect, although readily it leaves its heavy mark on brain development, will of course not be remembered.

Lisa was, at least most of the time, very protective of her mother, who had had a terrible childhood herself. Lisa seemed to prefer not to examine that relationship for quite a while. Certainly, in cases like this, we collect the data again, quietly. We can only surmise that attention and real care were little known (when most needed,) so what was never known, of course, will not be missed or expected, or understood. There is virtually no category for it in their psyches.

Eventually, they may become aware of judgment or anger, about neglect, at least sometimes, especially if a young child or baby in their lives might awaken the questions. For Lisa, it was several years in before she could wonder, "How could this have happened? She was home, never worked outside the house or even went anywhere. Where was she? I was a baby!"

This is the initial conundrum we must cautiously navigate. Our show of care may or may not be noticed; and if noticed may be disbelieved, mistrusted, or simply dismissed. Especially in this odd relationship that involves an exchange of money. Or perhaps placing value on our relationship, may seem to connote "weakness," an unbearable point of shame and vulnerability. If perceived at all, we may be more like an instrument, a surgical tool or an (it is hoped) skilled technician, even a bus driver whose task is to know the geography and just get them to their destination as quickly as possible: or a cloudy blob in a distant chair like my therapist was for an embarrassingly long time. We may be more like that, than an actual person like themselves. The therapist's mindful, thoughtful and non-defensive steady attention to this relationship is paramount.

The question then becomes, how do we make this early stage interesting and valuable? How do we begin to create traction, especially if the client is eager to see results, or to be done with it, or are still trying to decide if it is worth being there, or what they would see as results.

Howard had left a wake of brief and discarded therapists behind him, and was initially "shopping," which has not been unusual for me. To inquire as to why he chose not to continue with one of the past therapists, or why he came to me was and often is useful. In my case, because I am also a sex therapist, he chose me, both because he was confused and troubled by his own sexuality, but also that of Robin, his ex. He had not been able to get help with that from any of the others. Some come to me because they are intrigued by reading about Neurofeedback either on my website, or somewhere else, and few therapists around here offer it. Often the answers are much less substantive, and as arbitrary as location, or what time in my schedule might be open. Questions about prior therapists may bring a similar range of responses.

Beyond that, the primary through-line and centerpiece begins: our task is thoughtful, consistent and ever-mindful presence and interest in whatever may be of interest to them. Being a good listener, asking questions and staying with what is of greatest interest to them, which may or may not be of primary interest to us; tracking well, and remembering well. I have never been much for note taking, and relied on my steel-trap memory. But I anticipate a time when the old trap may lose its spring and I will need to write more down. There is no shame in that. It beats the alternative, and humility goes a long way.

Secure your knowledgeable and trusted consultant if you haven't already, because relying on more oblique transferences, especially when they may more than usual engage our own material, is essential. We definitely want to keep our own "stuff" out of it. If you can find someone who knows developmental trauma, even better. And one of the blessings of the Pandemic is how many webinars and conferences are now available online. So even for more "obscure" or less readily accessible content areas, good training can be had.

Sometimes this early stage can be hard to sit through. With Jim, whom we have yet to meet, the first year or two were as if he was under water with a mouth full of marbles. He seemed to have his own language, which I often could not comprehend, and his translations were often not much better. He had a unique vocabulary for both his somatic symptoms and his depression, and when I asked for more clarity, his responses were equally vague and metaphorical. The best I could do was to try and keep track and cobble together some sort of image or a special "Jim dictionary" which I imagine is what he always wished someone would do; while also attempting to understand the meaning of his being so opaquely unique. It was clear that he was also desperately trying to convince himself that he was authentically "ill" and not just a "jerk" but portraying himself as so different from the rest of the species, this took a while for me to grasp.

Coming from an Ivy League family, he needed to be seen as smart, perhaps smarter than me. I needed to demonstrate both that I was smart enough, but comfortable enough with not being smarter than he. Hearing his occasional commentary on Quantum Physics and Buddhism was such a challenge. His descriptions of childhood at this stage were similarly impressionistic, and peppered with dramatic angry diatribes, which included loud proclamations of "I don't want to be here!" meaning on this planet. He had never attempted suicide and did not intend to start now. But he needed to use that vehicle for expressing how utterly miserable, out of place and alone he felt in the world. And again, he needed me to accept his language.

When at his initial shopping stage, I asked why he chose me, Jim responded without hesitation, that it was because I offered the option of 90-minute sessions. He had not heard of that before and immediately knew it was for him. Early in the therapy, Jim began a routine, of spending sometimes 20 or 30 minutes at the start of each session in his own unique exercise routine, stretching and popping joints. I remember needing to vent quite at length with my ever-patient consultant, about how devalued and disrespected I felt. My task was to prove myself able to sit with all of that, and be present, to enter and respect his exquisitely unique personal world. It was not easy, but it was easier than what came later, which I will recount in its time. Jim generously and enthusiastically gave me carte blanche to write about our story. He was happy at the thought that he might be able to help others that way, and we both know he is a success story for us both. He is now not only proud but also grateful. But I get ahead of myself.

In this early stage, we quietly do what we do with all new clients, which is attempt to enter their world, which may be dramatically different like Jim's or some of the clients I have had who come from far away countries and cultures, or others like Jackie's which are so devoid of descriptors that the challenges of staying present are different.

## A "ONE PERSON PSYCHOLOGY"

My client Stan taught me much about what I came to refer to as a "one person psychology," which is a hallmark of neglect. Stan who grew up on a small European family farm. At first blush, it sounded picturesque and quaint to me, picturing the landscape of a European mountain town. It evoked favorite images from my childhood, Heidi, or The Sound of Music. But it really was not like that. Stan was another child saddled with a heavy responsibility of daily tasks well before school age. In his large family, everyone was perennially busy and efficiency and discipline were assumed and necessary. No one talked very much. As an adult, he was quite tall, and his wife Cora, was a tiny woman. His habit of storing essential, daily use household items like coffee or toilet paper on a very high shelf; or on a walk allegedly *with* her, walking faster on his long legs than she could possibly keep up with, were small things that perpetuated a redundant flood of complaints from her, that were a chronic annoyance to him. Their repetitive sequence about this, was like a rehearsed and tired musical "call and response." She simply could not understand how he could completely lose track or lose sight of her on their walks, even not notice for quite a while that she was unhappily many paces behind. He talked to himself some, even when she was around, and at least in her view, made decisions "like a single person." After decades of marriage, she was convinced that there was "something wrong with him." He was reminiscent of the immature, inconsiderate and selfish young guys she dated in college, not what she expected from a husband and father in his fifties. How did it happen that he could "forget" all about her? Or their two boys? Or be seemingly oblivious to her presence or absence?

Stan did not understand why Cora would make such a big deal of "little, insignificant things." Stan's world fit the description or the fitting term the "one-person psychology." The child of neglect can become quite unconscious and oblivious to the other's whereabouts or even existence, to varying degrees, just as they themselves fell out of the minds of their important caregivers, or perhaps were never in them to speak of, at all.

In Stan's childhood, no one looked out for him or even knew where he was or more importantly *who*, he was, as long as the work got done. On one hand, his parents were all powerful, and he was scrupulously aware of doing a "good job" and pleasing or displeasing them.

The inevitable consequences of a failure or misstep were serious enough that Stan became a vigilant observer and student of his parents' character and behavior, becoming a self-styled "expert" on them, at least in his own eyes. This also became his habit in the world. A focus outward; the belief that *the other has all the power*, and his own existence or value to anyone else, are all questionable in the interpersonal world. Stan adapted by going about his life, taking care of business and looking out for himself.

On the other hand, these same all-powerful parents rather resembled the invisible parents in the old *Peanuts* cartoon, or Columbo's wife. The reader/audience never sees them, so they are a mythical specter that exist somewhere in the background rather like props in the story, not real characters in it. They become cardboard cutout-like, as do many, many other people in these clients' lives. Including possibly, we therapists. We don't quite "exist" much as they often did not realize that they felt, at least in the interpersonal world.

I remember when I was in first grade in New York City. We were shopping at Kroger's and I was amazed to run into my teacher Miss Wiesjahn. I was stunned to see that she had a cart full of grocery items, butter, eggs, fruit and bread. I remember thinking with surprise, "Wow, Miss Wiesjahn eats food!" Much like my own therapist, we may readily take on that kind of hazy vagueness in their minds.

To some extent, this was Stan's wife's complaint about his view of her. She felt like an "object," and to some extent she was. And so are we, (which in some clinical language is what we are called.) In the world where Stan and Cora came of age, object and certainly "sex object" had a political cast, and "sex object," particularly insulted Stan. He had always treasured his sexual relationship with Cora, and really loved her. He was not only incensed but also hurt, although that would be a bit much for him to recognize.

"In spite of all that he did do, how could she possibly …?" After all, he dutifully, consistently, and scrupulously efficiently fulfilled his responsibilities as a good earner, a faithful spouse and loving father, at least in his own eyes. He could not understand what she wanted to "talk" about or what was "missing." He felt unseen, unappreciated and taken for granted for all the devotion and care that he did demonstrate, and "truly did not know what to do. There simply was nothing he could do!" the soon to be familiar refrains of the song of neglect.

Stan was a doer, and also an impassioned political activist. He was inflamed by political leaders who usurped or misused their power, and the lack of dignity, respect and care they showed for the "little guy." Stan could get very wrapped up and spend "huge" amounts of time on his political life, which Cora did not share. This was another of her chronic complaints, he was so busy, and busy in ways that again, made her feel superfluous, like she "did not occupy any real estate in his over-crowded head."

Apparently, no one had ever really missed him before. Stan's feelings readily showed themselves in his activism, and he could be highly emotional there. He knew he really loved his wife and he believed he was devoted in showing his care. He was frustrated that his efforts did not seem to register.

All in all, Stan viewed his life as "pretty darn good." His parents now elderly, were modest, well-intentioned, farm people and doting grandparents. He had done well and had no interest in mining for ways to find fault with them. Stan had precious little to say about his childhood and his family. Frankly, he did not really know why it might be relevant. The idyllic scenes were the story he knew and told. So, what's the problem?

The fatigue and frustration of the unending cycle of dialog, finally won him over to Cora's wish that they enter couples therapy. She had been agitating for it for a long time, and he finally "caved." He had really reached his limit with her criticism. It was only then, in our therapy, that Stan began to talk about his childhood, largely because my inquiry about it, was in the interest of helping Cora (and himself) make sense out of their differentness. The result was that he began to slowly connect more with his past and even his feelings, and Cora began to soften, which was for him a welcome incentive.

When the new term "social distancing" emerged with The Pandemic of COVID 19, Stan felt oddly copasetic with not only the concept but even the language, like comfy old slippers. The mandate to stay at home in quarantine, and minimally interact with anyone outside of our immediate households, only with face masks and at a physical distance of at least 6 feet was our reality for months on end. For Stan, and many a child of neglect, it was both a familiar and even "normal facsimile of their whole lives," with the exception that stores and restaurants were closed, and we were surrounded by fear and death. He said with a slight laugh, "I feel I spent my whole life training for this." This also irked Cora, and she was surprised when in a rare moment of candor he divulged a gnawing emptiness that seized him when he was not busy. This was news to her. Cora learned that his default, learned in childhood to ward off undesirable feelings, was to keep busy. On the farm, there was no time to notice his loneliness, anxiety and depression.

At school Stan had trouble with concentration and focus. If he were in grammar school now, he would have been tested for some sort of attentional problem. As it was then, he suffered silently and secretly from terrible difficulty reading; and lived in dread of circle time when going around the class and taking a turn at reading a section aloud. He would try to count paragraphs and figure out ahead which would be his segment, so he might to try to practice in advance. Usually he struggled painfully and haltingly to get through whatever it was, if he did not succeed in escaping to the bathroom to miss his turn. Terribly ashamed he would withdraw into silence until the next time. Stan never told his parents about this almost daily torment, in fact, he may have never told anyone before now. No one noticed and no one knew.

Stan became a good athlete, and particularly enjoyed baseball, which although it is a team sport, does not involve the close physical contact or more intense interdependence and interaction of some of the other sports. The camaraderie of the team, his success as a player, and the overall regulating effect of physical exercise became ways to manage his loneliness. But admittedly at times, he just felt "lost." When he discovered alcohol and other mood-altering substances as he got a little older, they offered a welcome solution. Here was yet another way of creating a protective barrier, against emotion from the inside, and unwanted "interruption" from them. Cora felt duly "banished." Stan disavowed interpersonal need early and out of necessity. Cora was left to wonder, where does that leave her? And where does that leave someone like a therapist?

It is a balancing act. Particularly with someone like Stan. We must be exquisitely present, in the way no one ever was, attentive to who the client is, track carefully and remember what they say. And yet remain unobtrusive, cautiously assume a role of caring without calling attention to ourselves. And we must tolerate the ambivalence they may feel about being there. With Stan for many months, I was weekly readily prepared for him to say he wanted to "take a break" meaning end therapy. He would routinely joke, "are we done yet?" Or lament the admittedly long drive to my office, (which Cora loved, as it was uninterrupted time with him). Or wanting to come less frequently because of the expense. It was nearly a year before I stopped wondering if they would "stick." The way I felt devalued and not good enough was a window into his chronic childhood experience of feeling just like that. He could not tell me about it in language, but inducing the feelings in me, he could *show* me. Again, stay attuned to all the various media and languages of nonverbal communication that these clients use to reveal the story.

Through understanding more about his own history, Stan was able to open to the loneliness of that busy, socially distant life on the farm. He began to recognize how the measure of his worth, even his identity itself, had been his productivity, what he could accomplish. He began to understand why he became so snappish or defensive when Cora, attempting to make friendly contact, would ask him "how was your day?" He heard in that, not a greeting, but an accounting or evaluation: "What did you accomplish today?" Now that made sense to both of them. And Cora learned that Stan needed to be seen and appreciated, once he figured out how that could be achieved. As Cora gradually softened, Stan slowly and cautiously allowed her to enter his formerly always one-person world. His awareness of her slowly widened, not without reminders of course, and not overnight. He was delighted (and his behavior was duly re-enforced) at how her complaining gradually diminished and virtually stopped.

## CHILDREN OF NARCISSISTS

Often the neglect is the result of having a narcissistic parent (or two!) The parent is so self-absorbed, grandiose, busy with their own achievements or persona in the world, that as I often point out to them "There is no you." The injury is profound. They may be on a desperate quest to earn the right to exist, or to discover what it takes to be worthy enough to merit the ground one inhabits on the earth. They may try perfectionism, overachievement, undying service to the world. They may endlessly struggle about being good enough, or what it takes to be wanted or worthy to take up space. They may be grandiose and somewhat narcissistic themselves, in their passion about "not being like that!" meaning the self-obsessed parent. They may have become enlightened to the diagnosis and literature both clinical and popular on Narcissism and "know it all." Most importantly they will be scrupulously vigilant for signs of it in us. We must be knowledgeable, prepared for and tolerate that, including suspicions or accusations, or simply assumptions of self-interest, and that we are not authentically interested in them. And we must be willing to look at ourselves dispassionately, honestly and with humility; and mine the rich vein of what they are telling us about their story. They may not yet know it.

   Some clients feel, more connected and appreciate therapist self-disclosure. For others it strikes the nerve of parental narcissism. Some are so accustomed to massaging the ego of the narcissistic parent, that they will lapse into the customary habit of inquiring even at length about the therapist, and then resenting it, or feeling eclipsed. I have been accused (of slipping and) talking too much, and admittedly at times it is true, and I must be more mindful.


## THE CHILD OF NEGLECT IN PARTNERSHIP

For many a child of neglect, couples therapy is the way they land in our offices. It is generally counter-intuitive and for many, highly unlikely for them to seek "help" for themselves. In my practice, many came with partners who had more visible or tangible problems or histories, like dramatic abuse and glaring presentations of PTSD. They wanted help "fixing" their partner. Often it was hard for them to speak of themselves at all, or they believed there was nothing important to tell. They might answer a question about themselves by going on at length about the partner or the partner's feelings, or even speak for the partner-if we let them. They might have an elaborate analysis of the partner that they are eager to relay to the therapist. Self-styled experts, they may seem to be almost playing therapist themselves. Perhaps they have read widely on what they think is the partner's problem. Their complaints and frustrations are about that or so they think.

When at first I take the time to try and know who *they* are, the attention may be unwelcome. They are not used to it, they don't like it, or they think it is irrelevant. It is also convenient for the partner to occupy the role of "problem child," which leaves them comfortably "off the hook." I always tell them straight away, that that model does not fly with me. One partner gets all the blame and all the help. The other is free of blame and responsibility, but doesn't get anything else either. And we all know it is really never true, that one partner in a dyad is the problem.

What I then have to listen for, is where the "charge" is about the partner. Whatever is most upsetting about the partner, will probably point us directly to the worst of the childhood pain. When the biggest upsets about the partner, are about feeling ignored, abandoned or unheard, that is informative. It may be a while before we learn where the pain is, and our inquiries or empathy are received. The therapist must expect to be dismissed, and build a thick skin to maintain warm and empathic attention. It may require much time, sometimes some sort of "breakthrough" event, before there is a shift in the attachment to the therapist. And even when there is, it may be fragile or temporal for a very long time, or even seem to vanish.

Couple's work is an opportunity to see the client's attachment behavior live, from the outside, and in relation to someone who in most cases, truly matters to them. It may also be a first experience of having an advocate, someone to see and help them see what they are trying to communicate, and unaware of. They crave to be seen and heard, and often are not in contact with what it is they are desperate to communicate, or how incomplete, vague, non-verbal, sparse or inaudible their expressions are. The therapist who is able to slow things down enough to notice, ask, attempt to "translate" into a form that the spouse can hear is invaluable. In spite of themselves the child of neglect begins to perk up like a parched plant. And the partner who has been craving connection from "heart" is infinitely more drawn to them, more generous and interested. Then with luck, their most profound need which is to feel *wanted* begins to occur. This is what we strive for and it is a great day, if they stay long enough.

Presence, advocacy, consistency, equal and steady attention, authentic care, are all profoundly important. I can't emphasize this enough. If successful, we make an important mark on the attachment system. I have not infrequently had the experience where long after the couples work is over and past, even many years later, the child of neglect returns for some sort of individual work. They may trust that we know them well enough, and even remember their story enough to continue the journey, with us. It is often very rewarding for us both, and we may be surprised to learn that we therapists have remained an important icon of attachment and safety, in their internal worlds. I generally tell these clients when they leave, including when they leave what I at least, might consider "prematurely," "You are always welcome here. This is a 'life membership.'" (Except in the rare instance, of course, when they are not.)


## THE PROBLEM OF "THREES"

A parting point, or closing alert about couple's therapy with neglect, is a dynamic I call, "the problem of threes." One of the multiple advantages of couple's therapy, is that it can replicate a family type group. There will be many occasions where the therapy room will feel homey, cozy and intimate. This is most often when we are making headway and gaining harmony as a team. At other times, in our little group, a warm and fuzzy climate is not present at all, most likely depending both on how we are doing, but also or depending on the precise nature of the neglect history of the client.

Elaine came from a large family, in which she was the second to the youngest child. She also happened to be of a culture that devalued girls, so she was doubly lost in the crowd. She often accused me, not only of siding with her partner. Vanessa, who was white and blond, and particularly attractive. Vanessa wore colorful and beautiful clothes, was flamboyant, and arguably "sexy." Elaine certainly thought so. But even worse, because Vanessa was white and blond, and younger. Elaine was convinced that I "preferred Vanessa's blond hair and blue eyes."

As a couples' therapist I strive to be equidistant and view both partners equally. (Not always easy as we all know, when some clients truly are much easier to like.) And more personally as a politically and socially motivated human being who also happens to be the child of two Holocaust survivors, I struggled against being shocked, offended, incensed and at the very least horrified by the persistent accusation. Especially as I was working so hard to help the couple work through the recurrent theme of jealousy in their relationship.

Elaine was perpetually suspicious of Vanessa, of having designs on, or of infidelity with others, even men in whom Vanessa had unquestionably "*zero* interest!" As is now familiar to us, Elaine was adamant and immovable from "knowing" what she knew. Even when it was about Vanessa, or in this case about me. She loudly and unequivocally "saw what she saw, and knew what she knew!"

In Elaine's family, absolutely everything was in short supply. Her single mother with a large brood, was already exhausted and depleted by the time Elaine was even born. She felt unwanted from the start. And there was not enough money, not enough space, not enough food, and most of all, not enough love or attention. Elaine was ever keenly aware of who got what and how much. And the boys were unabashedly favored. As hard as Elaine had tried, from the beginning of her life, she could not make her mother "happy," and could not seem to win her attention, care or love. I felt similarly in my tireless efforts with her.

It is not always easy to hold the big picture when we are being devalued and ragefully bashed, or accused. In fact, there are times when the therapist is hard pressed to contain the projection and might be too infuriated to discern the message of the projective identification. Admittedly I felt that way at times with Elaine. It may become clear only later, after the session, when I was able to calm down and disentangle the information about Elaine from all the noise, both my own and hers.

Elaine had ever suffered excruciatingly from extreme jealousy whenever she was in any grouping larger than a dyad. She always expected to be ignored, disliked or simply to vanish whenever there was more than herself and one other, in any mix. Attentive like a hawk, for rejection or double standards, she was astutely and quickly able to fabricate a detailed fiction of evidence, often in sophisticated clinical language. She lost many relationships this way, which was her greatest agony. It was what she was attempting to incite help with, in this very primitive way. Better with me than Vanessa. My challenge was to stay as non-defensive and compassionate as humanly possible.

The expectation to be rejected or simply disappear from the awareness of the other, most decidedly including the therapist, is a not uncommon sequela of neglect. Threes, can arguably be a known challenge, even under ordinary and non-clinical circumstances, and with just anyone really, as with the old adage I remember from grammar school "Two is company, three is a crowd," which was sadly always true for me. It may make couples therapy with neglect survivors extra challenging in some cases, or even contraindicated before more work has been done on the neglect individually.

In the preferable case, it can be highly adaptive, and a resourceful and effective use of the therapist, to shift the transference, and the focus in this way. Clients may utilize us in this manner with other issues as well, as a vehicle for communicating the story that is not known or has no words, yet. For the therapist it may be no fun at all. Again, reliable, knowledgeable and safe consultation is of the essence, good self-care and careful scheduling so as not to have too many such clients in one day!

## SUMMING UP AND WHAT TO DO

- Presence is the single most important part of our task, which makes its vehicle, the therapeutic relationship, extremely important. It is where we can have the most impact, (positive or negative I might sadly add).

- We must be ever mindful and attuned to what the therapeutic relationship communicates or attempts to communicate about early attachment, including the non-verbals: enactments, body language, tone that is incongruent with content, and feelings inside the therapist that strangely don't feel like one's own. We may not always be able to speak of them with the client, but to notice and make use of them as we can.

- Parental narcissism may be a variation of neglect that is not immediately obvious, to the client, or to us. The parent may have been so intrusive, that it is not apparent how utterly absent they were to the client. It may be most clearly expressed in the therapeutic relationship, and come to light in that way, if we are paying attention.

- Couples therapy can be a very effective modality for working with neglect. In the best of circumstances, it can be very family like, and the therapist is in a positive and protective caregiver role. The therapist can observe the attachment interactions and patterns live and from the outside. And I always say and continue to believe: nothing takes us so directly to core attachment material like the intimate partnership. So, it can be invaluable. Also, clients can readily shift the projections to the therapist, which both makes us a vessel for powerful projective identification, and information about their early attachments. Having the partner both witness and empathize, as well as see and learn about them, can forge growing attachment with both self and the partner.
- Similarly, the projections can be deeply challenging for the therapist.
- Groupings of three, such as the couple's therapy, can be a setting where jealousy and scarcity tendencies emerge. We must be both watchful for this, if we can see it coming. And (in an exceptionally small number of cases in my experience,) couples therapy may be contraindicated until more individual therapy on the neglect, has been done.
- Therapist humility is paramount. We must have the willingness to listen and self-correct; apologize when our attunement misses the mark, or when our perception is unsatisfactory to them, which may be often. Or when our expressions of care don't land well. I had one client who said that sometimes when he cried, and I made what to me might be comforting or empathic sounds, (often that I was not fully aware of,) he experienced it as pity and found it humiliating. He felt pathetic, "pitiful" and weak. I had to be mindful to cut that out. To own and apologize for missteps, is powerful and among their sorely missing experiences.
- Patience with their impatience. This can be no small feat and may inspire didactic or theoretical questions, and debates of what "works" including their avowed expertise gleaned from the internet, their friends, or pop psychology. Again, humility and openness are of the essence, especially when it feels particularly insulting to the therapist. It also means being confident, prepared and transparent about one's approach, and

about what we believe is effective and why. Often these people are extremely smart and well read. They certainly want to know that we know what we are doing. And often they have bitter previous therapy experiences. Some clients are interested in didactic explanations. Others find them boring, or just float off. Again, staying present and attuned is our best guide.

- Because of their self-reliance and fierce attachment to what they "know" it is important to maintain one's authority as the therapist and the one directing the therapy, being flexible and open to input, and still remaining true to one's own expertise (and short-comings) and boundaries. Ironically, they will feel safer knowing there is someone there to contain them, even if they rebel against it. They never had a caregiver strong enough or present enough to withstand and keep them safe as they defined themselves and discovered their own power.

- Again, bring your whole body and psyche to the work with them, given their many different languages of expression. Unquestionably many children of neglect will be vigilant to all of it. This means remaining mindful as to how we organize the workday; being well rested; well-nourished; and well-regulated oneself! It is always essential to keep the instrument tuned!

## BIBLIOGRAPHY

Spyri, Johanna. *Heidi*. Adapted by Deirdre S. Laiken. New York: Baronet Books, 2008. First published 1880 by Justus Perthes (Gotha, Germany).

Tatkin, Stan. "Allergic to Hope: Angry Resistant Attachment and a One-Person Psychology within a Two-Person Psychological System." *Psychotherapy in Australia* 18, no. 1 (November 2011): 30–37.

Wise, Robert. *The Sound of Music*. Beverly Hills, California: Twentieth Century Fox, 1965.

# Chapter 4

# "But Nothing Happened to Me!": What's the Story?

Another challenge of our work, stems from clients' confused and sometimes even angry insistence that they have "no story." Where some might not even notice or think about it, others searching for a traumatic, or some kind of explanation for the difficulties or unhappiness they experience, come up empty. When invited to explore, they may come to the defense of parents whom they may admire, idealize or pity. This may make sense, as in many cases parents had their own trauma history, and/or poverty, war, racism or their own childhood abuse, for example, or if parents were simply and desperately trying to make ends meet, and for that reason unavailable, preoccupied, troubled or absent.

Many neglect clients don't remember much about their childhoods at all, a common adaptation. The therapist must be painstakingly tactful, cautious, respectful and creative to uncover the story and make use of it. This is a key process and an ongoing one in the work with these people. And if like Jim, not having a story to point to, and an "excuse" for the sorry state of my life, just means "I'm a jerk," an all the more delicate one. Clients may stay attached to the "jerk" hypothesis, or whatever theirs might be, which may in itself be another hint about their past. At this point, we want to take our time and just notice and track for these points of heightened emotion which will be informative about unremembered story.

Once we have begun to identify or at least suspect that neglect is the issue, and set about the task of building a relationship and entering a historically private world, we learn where the client themselves estimate the "presenting problem" to be. As we now know, they themselves may not be so sure, which may in itself be a clue. As with any psychotherapy client, we meet the client where they are. However, I will add that being story-less is rather like floating rudder-less, lost and adrift. Narrative is key to a coherent sense of self, and feeling anchored. The feeling that comes with story-lessness may very well replicate the "at sea" experience of the neglected child, especially when they are very young.


## BEGINNING WITH THE STORY THEY BRING

Randi came to therapy because she could not understand why her grief and tears about a short, failed relationship, were so profound, protracted and unrelenting. She had been virtually immobilized with sadness, confusion and loss for two years already, and she still could not stop herself from going to Facebook to find out what she could about the lost lover, which only invariably made her feel worse, and more self-deprecating. She might spend hours staring at herself in the mirror, sometimes with and other times without clothes, trying to see what he saw or did not see, trying to "figure it out." She just couldn't, and she just couldn't let go of it. Was she too ugly, too fat, boring, stupid, not sexy enough, too old, or all of the above? It could only be some fatal flaw in her, as her assumption in general: *everything* was *always* her fault. Coming from a "one-person-psychology" orientation, there will be no other explanation.

Because there is no other, the child of neglect will feel responsible for everything. I remember one client who had desperately wished to contract cancer, or some dreaded disease, or *something* that would not be his "fault," that might get someone to care. But even cancer he would have found a way to blame himself for. I like to tell people early on in the therapy, that mine is a "no-fault paradigm." I believe there is never only one responsible party in any relationship. There is *always* a shared onus when things do not go well.

However, there is one exception of course, which is infant and parent. In that case, the parent is *fully* responsible. Infants and children do not have the sufficiently developed mental and physical equipment, to be responsible, and it is quite a while before they do. With the same being true in the therapist client dyad, which in effect replicates the parent-child relationship. The child of neglect is most likely so accustomed to a default to self-blame, that they cannot make use of this. Like many things, it is something we will have to repeat often, and attempt to demonstrate. As ever, there is a lot for us both to take in early in a therapy, so as therapists, we must choose our timing judiciously, and listen carefully.

Randi was not able to listen to much just yet, and had never really recounted the whole story of the relationship. So at least a part of her was eager to do so, if also apprehensive to reveal herself that much. But she urgently wanted to understand what had happened so she could learn from it, and so she could find a life partner. That she desperately wanted. She was 33, her biological clock was loudly ticking, and she longed to have a family. Of course, I had my theory early on about her childhood antecedent, but talking about child-hood was clearly not her interest, or apparent need.

Randi and I spent months slowly combing the story of the lost relationship. It was clearly a relief to her, to unburden herself about it for the first time. She brought an accumulated wealth of detail, that included collected text messages, emails and photos, in addition to her exacting and copious memory. It was painful for her, but as we slogged through it, she did notice that her sleep improved slightly and she was perhaps "a little bit" less obsessed than she had been before we began. I suspected that was due to just having some empathic other in there with her, especially as I learned about how solitary and lonely her life since the break-up had been and still was; and really always had been for that matter. She was most eager to examine what her part had been, preferring not to vilify Richard, her ex. She told me repeatedly she did not want me to be too "soft" on her. She so wanted to learn from her mistakes, and not repeat them.

It must have been at least five painstaking months, that we spent reviewing the story. Once she had "gotten it all out," she seemed to want to just jump into whatever was next. Almost as if it were con-fession, where all she really had to do was say it all to another human being. She collapsed into the familiar "I don't know" or "I don't know what to do" mode. I asked her, "what would you like from me around this?" She finally did have an answer, she did have a role for me.

Randi wanted me to be a kind of Wikipedia of information about relationship. Having heard the story, she wanted to know what I thought she "should" have done differently. I was able to point to how the "one-person psychology" aspect of her nature might have worked against her, not using those words of course. Richard may have felt unconsidered, or experienced her focus on work, her own travel and projects, as frustrating or simply distasteful. And to me both she and Richard seemed timid and ambivalent about sex. Perhaps he was as inexperienced as she was, and both were trying to conceal that. And they were unable to really talk about it. To me, Richard sounded young and non-committal, and pretty insecure himself, but she really only wanted to look at her own part, which I did honor.

However, Randi continued to be mystified as to why she just could not get over him, why she could not move on and even look at someone else. She would log onto the dating apps, and then find herself in tears, and just turn the phone off. As humiliated as she was about losing him, she still pined and longed for him to come back. After nearly six months, she asked me what I thought about that. Then I was able to ask her about her childhood.

Randi began to recount bits and pieces of the story that she only knew from what she had been told, or what she had learned from old fading black and white photos. Randi's mother had left her to be raised by an aunt before she was a year old. Her aunt had been rather cold, busy and had several small children of her own. Randi only remembered being an outsider in that family.

The explanation had always been that her mother had to go to work and earn in the big city, she was young and single and doing what she believed to be best for her little daughter. Randi never saw her mother much, her memory was minimal, but in later conversations, her aunt told her that she had been a quiet and solitary toddler. In the photos she showed me, I saw a sweet little girl with the most heartbreakingly sad and forlorn eyes and droopy posture. She did remember gaining weight and become depressed in adolescence, but she had never correlated the loss of her mother to the later snowballing difficulties that seemed always to constellate around some sort of abandonment. She had always really believed that her mother did the best she could, and what seemed to be best for her child.

Randi became interested in reflecting on her mother and her childhood, and beginning to process more of what she did and did not know; what she was and was not able to find out from relatives. It did not immediately resolve her relationship grief about Richard, but it made sense to her and helped her to feel less pathological. And she felt perhaps a wee bit empowered that all this grief might be about more than Richard. She did not want to think he alone had that much of a hold on her. And it gave us a direction and a focus for our subsequent work. Little by little he began to fade. She settled in to exploring her childhood and her history, and what it could tell her about herself. And she was keen on trying neurofeedback to work with material too early to remember.

Slowly and quietly I had to follow her lead. There were more than a few times I had to apologize for taking issue with some of Richard's behavior. She needed to get to the anger herself, which she did. And she even gradually became able to touch the edges of her anger at her mother, whom she had always sympathized with and defended.

For others, teasing out the childhood story may be even more of a challenge. They may feel so strongly about the recent event, that they don't want to diminish or invalidate it by doing what I might view as taking it deeper. Or they might feel unheard. "You don't understand! I am upset about *this*!" We must be patient, understanding and flexible, and as with Randi, work with their "schedule" even if they simultaneously are impatient with us.

After enough recounting and processing of childhood antecedents, and experiencing the resulting shift and relief, Randi did become more curious and interested in making more connections. I felt freer to talk about neglect, and she wanted to know more. In general, as the process of filling in the gaps in narrative advances, clients begin to experience change in their lives. In Randi's case she felt calmer and more confident, as the obsession with Richard slowly resolved. She was not quite ready to meet someone, but she felt more hope.

Again, we do this by following the access route of what is most available. In Randi's case, it was the grief about Richard, as in the couple's work it would be the most recent round of heavy conflict between the partners. Randi could not remember her mother actually leaving, but she could remember little flashbulbs about being in her aunt's family, that brought waves of tears, that felt very similar to the tears about Richard. She remembered the feelings of rejection by her cousins, and wondering "what is wrong with me?!" much as she had relentlessly felt for the last two years. Working back from what is most available, we wait. Clients will show greater or lesser reluctance to make this exploration. The therapist needs to get "comfortable" and again flexible and patient with the asking, the waiting and the frequent "pushback."


## WHY NARRATIVE MATTERS

I remember maybe 25 years ago in one of my survivor groups, there was a woman in the group who was a talented graphic artist. As a birthday gift she made for Louann, one of the other group members, a large and beautiful, colorful wall hanging that said in bold artistic letters: "Louann Matters!" One of the terrible sequelae of Louann's abuse history, was the Greek chorus in her head of "I don't matter," a not unusual default when trauma and/or neglect have occurred.

At the time of this writing, our world is erupting with questions about who and what "matters." The recently emerging Black Lives Matter movement is appropriately and at long last, placing the question squarely in our awareness. For now over two centuries, our African American population has lived that same reality, and been haunted by the same chorus, and had not only their dignity and freedom but also virtually any defining sense of self stripped away. Reduced to the role of object, tool, instrument of labor, or even worse beast of burden, identity was ravaged and pillaged. And although some of the forms of this have changed some, not nearly enough. It has still not stopped.

One impetus, dating back even to the long past days of the Civil Rights Movement, has been the endeavor of knowing and reclaiming personal and collective history, and naming clearly how it was mutilated, diluted, forgotten or rewritten. Knowing one's own story and truly owning it, being able to recount it and relay it to others; bequeathing it to generations that follow, erecting monuments, memorials and archives are a theme in the larger human story, and tremendously meaningful. Story is intrinsically tied to identity, to existence, and to a sense of self. These are enormous questions, and far beyond the scope of this book on childhood neglect.

In the brain, when the Default Mode Network, the web of circuitry that mediates sense of self is disconnected, meaning essential parts of the network are not making contact with other of the essential parts, the result is dullness, flatness, lack of aliveness. Ruth Lanius' lab has disturbing and illuminating data and neuro-imaging photos that demonstrate this impact of trauma and neglect. Story matters.

Perhaps the most powerful exposition I have seen yet of this complexity, is Ta-Nehisi Coates' first work of fiction, *The Water Dancer*, perhaps my favorite book of the decade. In expanding on it here, I do *not in any way* intend to dilute or detract from the unique and urgent matters facing our African American population, but rather to validate its significance. What matters to us, keenly affects identity, values and certainly behavior. Our world is forcing us to face this.

In Coates' story, the protagonist has a fractured identity, being the biological son of the white plantation-owner, in the antebellum south, and a young Black slave. His mother is sold away when he is an infant, so his story is a foggy haze. The boy is extraordinarily bright, unlike his obnoxious, "legitimate" white half-brother whose servant or "boy," he becomes. His father is proud of the protagonist's extraordinary brightness, and claims and showcases his talents, but on the other hand, cannot quite embrace him as a son. He is not white or "legitimate." So, he lives and grows up in a confused in between, not knowing his story or his mother; not really belonging anywhere; enjoying his intellectual gifts, but because he is not free, being unable to realize them. Freedom becomes his quest at all costs. Simultaneously, freedom interplays with love, attachment, identity, and the knowing of his story. Coates magnificently depicts why story matters so much, and why the neural networks mediating sense of self light up when it comes online.

The wisdom of the literature of social justice notwithstanding, the child of neglect might still wonder, who cares? What difference does it make now? Or because nothing remarkable seems to have occurred, there is really nothing to excavate. It can be a hard sell, especially if it seems to them to be a witch hunt or a search for skeletons. Important tasks for the therapist, are to make sure it does not become that; and to be clear about why it is important. Even if for a while, and sometimes quite a while, we must just hold that knowledge and not explicitly make use of it, we can hope that our interest and curiosity will inspire the same in them, and it often does.

Trauma of all sorts interrupts, disrupts and shatters the formation of coherent personal narrative, both by disorganizing the customary physiology of memory consolidation, and sheer confusion. The result can be a chaotic or spotty sense of self, and the host of accompanying affects and moods. Van der Kolk and Lanius have written and spoken eloquently on this. The "quieter" attachment trauma of neglect is no exception, and may be insidious because it is so often invisible even to children of neglect themselves. Narrative matters because it shapes and makes sense of who we are, and present ourselves to be. And again, bear in mind, the therapist's interest and curiosity about the story may or may not be welcome, certainly at first.

I might also add, that for many of these people, their appearance of success may be a foil, or at best double edged. They might look like a "success story." On one hand, this may be a welcome and prized protection against shame, "pity" and grief or anger; but it may also deceive the outside world such that no one knows the suffering, and the need for help or care, goes un-noticed, eliciting neglect, yet again. We must guard against making that mistake.

My client Frank experienced this mixed blessing through much of his life. His great professional success and multiple, expensive properties, made a stunning impression for his young years. And was also in some ways deceptive. Frank could rarely access deep emotion or memory and had only begun uncovering the tip of his neglect story when his little son turned five. Then he found himself feeling strangely moved by the special father-son time they spent together, reading books, putting together puzzles, making strawberry pancakes or building models. He cherished this time.

Frank began to notice that strangely, these precious times brought grief and sometimes even anger. It was like the old Polaroid snap shots, where slowly the image develops and the blur begins to emerge and come into focus. Slowly he began to see and remember wishing his Dad would spend time like this with him. He remembered spending virtually all of his time alone in his room, reading, often books remarkably beyond his age level. And he began to gain weight, and became the fat and ostracized child at school. All of this went un-noticed.

"I was a whiz kid academically, which also doesn't make a kid popular." Frank suffered with his weight and feeling ugly. "My dad might have noticed that I did well in school. But I never would have known it. I guess it was sort of expected. Nobody saw how I was blowing up into a butter ball, even though I kept needing bigger clothes. Sometimes I even had to try and get by in clothes that were clearly too small, because my mom didn't see or didn't get around to going shopping.

I remember just one time that he played catch with me. It stands out because I remember thinking 'wow, this has never happened before!' loving it and hoping it would happen again. It never did. The idea that he could feel the kind of delight spending time with me, that I feel with my kid, well it is unimaginable."

It is not unusual for a client who is a parent, to begin to recall imagery, memory and emotion, inspired by their own child. This can also help with the tendency toward minimizing the impact of their own experience, to imagine how they would feel if their own child felt like that. Then the empathic wave evokes compassion and contact, with a split off part of the self. As they experience the recovery of fragments of story, they feel more whole. Frank's mood, long a gnawing issue, began improving.

After this, I was able, through the therapy, to reference Frank's son, when he seemed to lack compassion or patience for himself, which became less necessary as he began to do that more for himself. As his son grew older, he enjoyed their time together even more, and was also able to feel proud of himself as a good dad, and that he was breaking the intergenerational chain. He was clearly convinced of the value not only to himself, of knowing and owning his story.

Pam, who had made a whole life of other-directedness and care-taking of others, was most aware of guilt and shame about growing up with wealth and privilege. Growing up in a small community of the highly educated, high-end elite was a chronic source of unworthiness. She believed she just had "too much money." Her depression made no sense to her, and she censured herself to be more grateful and to do more for the world. Her self-talk was vicious and unrelenting. The running narrative, brutal and exhausting and all my inner resources as an endurance athlete were required to ultimately penetrate it. I could barely fathom what it was like for her.

What we ultimately pieced together, over a very long run, was that Pam was the only child of a seriously narcissistic mother who was so demanding and so prescriptive of who Pam could *be*, as to crowd out the awareness of anything else. In her case, the poverty of mirroring was to the point of annihilation and truly felt deathly to her. And the voices were so loud, as to make any other part of her story inaudible for a long, long time. She knew only self-hatred and judgment for feeling so dead. She was an "ingrate!" And after all, she "had it all."

Pam was a long-term client, and for a long time, all I could do was mirror and empathize, mirror and empathize, and listen, not knowing if anything made any impression at all, least of all little bits of reflection about narcissism and neglect. Until one day Pam surprised me. In relief she exclaimed, "I would like to have a handicapped placard for my car, that says 'Child of Neglect!'" Her identity grew far beyond that initial discovery, but discovering her own neglect resulting from her mother's narcissism, was like a starting gun for her evolution and her healing.

Her mother's narcissism also confused and contaminated Pam's natural and profound longing to be truly seen. The abject poverty of mirroring, juxtaposed to her mother's hideously and coercively requiring Pam's and everyone's undying attention, complicated her balancing and understanding how much acknowledgment it is "OK" to want. Emerging from invisibility illustrated to her both how unseen she had always felt, and the depth of loneliness in that. But it also raised identity questions about what extent of "not wanting to be taken for granted" or wanting anything for herself, might signify a dreaded narcissism gene. In this regard, the therapist beyond the role of being a scrupulous and communicative mirror, must educate.

Pam also eventually was able to feel grateful for having enough money to come to therapy as much as she wanted or needed to. She also could see the immeasurable value to her own children of doing her personal work. She could use her money to do good works and to fund and support humanitarian projects and causes, and actually as she emerged from the echo chamber in her head, became increasingly politically and socially aware for the first time, and motivated to "be of use" by heart, and not driven by guilt and fear.

The elaboration of narrative is in essence the Michelangelo unearthing of the sculpture concealed in the rock. The sculpture already exists in there. We have "merely" to chip away at the layers of crusty sediment that conceal it. What does this mean concretely? Is presence, waiting and listening all we can do? Isn't there anything else? Well, if we are clear that neglect is the issue, to hold to an unwavering clarity about that. If there are points at which we can reference it or even educate about it without it sounding disjunctive or ax-grinding, I do. If an attachment image comes up in my mind, which it sometimes does, or a song, I might share that. Sometimes these seemingly random, momentary flashes are meaningful. Other times, they fall flat. We work with what the client presents first, as we did with Randi, for as long as it takes, and similarly with Pam, and everyone else. If we both stay the course, the story will find its way. And no, chipping away of rock is no walk in the park!

## BECOMING MULTI-LINGUAL: THE DIALECTS OF NEGLECT

My bias has always been realism in virtually all things. I like hard edged representational art; give me Diego Rivera over abstract or even Impressionist art. I prefer prose to poetry, just tell me outright what you mean so I don't have to figure it out. I prefer music with words, I've never cared for science fiction or fantasy because I can't quite believe it enough to be taken by the story. I have been challenged by cheesemaking because in addition to crucial and measurable temperatures, times and quantities, it is the world of nuance that makes for interesting and complex flavors. So, I must learn and practice this new world of sensory communication, which is often how story emerges. This has been a steep and rewarding learning curve for me!

The frontier of neglect can be a silent world. Solitude and minimal verbalization might be status quo. The child's experience might be that *no one is there* to listen, or no one really wants to know, so the default is to speak little, without awareness that it is little. Or to use verbalization to entertain or educate, to be of service. Whichever the variation, in order to help discover narrative, the therapist must cultivate fluency in a range of often challenging media.

The testimony of the body has been well described in the trauma literature. It may be another way that the story expresses itself. It is not always easy to interpret, and sometimes it is via symptoms that insist on attention in their own right. To try and see beyond them, if we don't do justice to them per se, may be experienced as yet another "failure to see." Caution is required in what we say aloud, but we can certainly be thinking metaphorically all the time, of the body as purveyor of the story. And somatic methodologies, as we will see in Chapter 10, are an essential component of our work. I strongly recommend incorporating them either oneself, which is preferable, or making reliable and skilled referrals.

Besides somatic symptoms, which are many, habits regarding food and sleep; effort and rest; even the sports these clients might choose or don't may be windows into the unremembered story. We have already seen a number of examples of dysregulated eating in the stories thus far, and the hint, that food was a comfort or companion when there was no other. I have also seen eating disorders on the other end of the spectrum. For example, Rachel, a child of a Holocaust survivor like me, grew up hearing her father bellow, "You don't know what it is like to go to bed hungry!" Rachel's anorexia was a way both to try and be like him, or be worthy enough to garner his attention by recreating his experience, in effect being like him. "Except it did not work. It was my fault. He was a victim and a hero. I was just bad."

For other anorexia and bulimia survivors the story has been about powerlessness, or never being good enough. Trying to have control over something, or be thin enough to please, may be another example of the story communicated through the body. We cannot, however, skip over the concrete to the metaphorical. My experience with eating disorders has been that most often, they are in the past and not acute when the client reaches me. But I don't work with teens or adolescents, so that may explain it. Again, good and specialized training and/or good referrals are of the essence here. And we maintain a watchful and thoughtful attention to the symptom, and hold in mind the question of what it may be trying to tell us.

I have been struck by the many endurance or "ultra" distance athletes with neglect histories I have seen. Alice was avid in the cycling sport of Randonneuring. She had more than a handful of times completed the famed Paris-Brest-Paris event which involved 1,200 grueling km (about 745 miles) in a 90-hour time limit, largely without sleep. She recounted with a laugh "I would just say to myself, 'Either it will get easier, it will end, or I will die! And it always did.'" The perseverance, pain, determination, strength, silence and extreme of self-reliance were a perfect metaphor for her lonely childhood. The sporting events were both a way for her to feel empowered and proud, as well as a vehicle of communication about her childhood world. We want to show interest in both. And inquiring about the metaphor, especially with someone like Alice, who loved talking about her sport, was both effective in reconstructive narrative, as well as building our relationship.

Ralph was a rock climber who showed me photos of the walls of smooth vertical stone where he might spend whole days scaling minute distances and creating a safe landing place for each foot before taking any step; sleeping in cold and unimaginably precarious nooks and crannies. As a child, no one ever really knew where Ralph was sleeping, that he was growing hallucinogenic mushrooms under his bed and roaming the country following a popular rock band before hitting his teens. By age 14, he had a full-on drug problem which did make him finally visible. None of this was noteworthy to him. And his drug recovery was another arduous and painstaking climb which he navigated successfully, with only his own "ropes and pitons" and without the more customary supports.

Now in his middle forties, living alone, successfully but solitary in his profession, he feared dipping into  the crippling depression of his twenties. And relationship was endlessly trying for him. But the inquiries about his climbs were an opportunity to know more about his story. His parents *now* having no idea that he was setting unprecedented records in his sport, which occupied large amounts of his time and interest, became a vehicle for remembering, and even feeling something about how unknown and forgotten he had always been.

I have learned to slowly and carefully ask for more information. Most often these clients have never really known or thought that anything about themselves might be unique or noteworthy. For some the ultradistances were initially a way of putting miles between themselves and what might have been a too-lonely, or confining environment. It was for me, in my discovery that running marathon distances before I was 12, made me feel free, accomplished and triumphant in my solitude; and seemed to get me "away." (And the activity may be another method of self-regulation; of managing a hyper-aroused or hypo-aroused nervous system.) We must go with great caution to not pathologize what may be a point of pride and pleasure, and self-regulation. As with many other "data points," we may need to hold and file our thoughts for some later time when interpretation might be more interesting, and thus helpful and welcome.

Another impressive and often baffling medium is the dissociated communication of enactment, where life or even the therapy itself becomes a theater for the unconscious. Most dramatically, we ourselves may unwittingly be cast into role. Especially if loss or abandonment occurred through the birth of one or more siblings; the chronic "competition" with a special-needs sibling; perhaps the parent's attention was compelled by some other relationship, be it the other parent or another partner and was therefore very absent due to that preoccupation. The jealousies can be vicious. Knowing we even have other clients may be enough to cast us into role.

One horrible experience, I can only interpret in this way. I still shudder to remember it, and am by no means using enactment as a way of explaining away or excusing what I did. However, it was a powerful communication of bitterly painful life experience that I have never forgotten, although it happened now many years ago. Fred was an extremely intelligent retired attorney, depressed and feeling stuck in his marriage and his life. He had the earmarks of neglect and seemed to soak up attention and a receptive ear, like a parched plant. He was likable and we seemed to make a good connection. I saw him off and on over a period of several years. He never stayed too long at one time, but for the most part, our stints were productive and enjoyable for both of us.

Fred felt bitterly frustrated and rejected by his wife. He always felt sidelined by their kids even now that they were all grown. He was chronically dissatisfied, feeling basically ignored by her, yet he could never quite give up on her. His cycling returns to therapy were usually when his frustrations got the better of him.

What I knew of Fred's childhood, was not too much. I did know that his mother preferred girls, or that is how he had always felt, and from the time his sister was born, something had changed. I did not quite get it, however, or he most certainly *felt* that I did not. Additionally, his memory reflected both his age, and the spottiness that neglect survivors so often have about their past. I tried to collect information about his childhood, but that mostly was not what he was interested in talking about, preferring to vent about his marriage. He found neurofeedback helped a lot with his depression, so often we did not even talk.

Because of his unstructured schedule as a retired person, Fred often needed to bounce around with his appointment times, which is not ordinarily how I work. On this particular day, when I came out to the waiting room to greet him, I was met by a therapist's worst nightmare. For the first and only time in my thirty-five years of practice, I had double booked. I was aghast. The woman whose regular appointment time I had offered to Fred, had canceled for not that week but the following. I had canceled the wrong week. What was I going to do? I am sickened to even remember this. I had no other times open that day or even that week. I gave the woman her hour and told Fred I would call him. He quietly left.

When I called him, he did not answer. He did not call me back. When I emailed him my profuse apology, there was no response. When I refunded a payment from his previous bill, again, no acknowledgment. I began to comprehend his heartbreak about being ever the unchosen one. And yet again, displaced or kicked aside for the "girl." I never saw Fred again. After several more attempts at contact I honored his clear wish to be done with me. I am deeply sad that I learned too late, but I hope that by sharing our story here, others will be spared.

I have often interpreted enactments aloud to couples, to help them comprehend each other's otherwise incomprehensible behaviors. It is an intense and effective medium of conveying particularly emotion that is often beyond words. Surely Fred's childhood pain was. Our takeaway is to be again, exquisitely mindful of oneself, perhaps more than ever, knowing that the communications about story take many and sometimes mysterious forms.

Had Fred returned, of course, we would begin with my authentic ownership and remorse for the injury and the mistake that did come from me. To hop over the concrete into the symbolic, would be yet another experience of ignoring or dismissing his feelings in our relationship, when that is fully processed, and it is hoped, healed, is when we can connect the dots to his mother and sister, but not too fast. Most importantly, to describe in fine detail the emotions I felt, that I can imagine were a window into his, then and now, so he finally feels like someone gets it. A piece of the story is now known. Then, the enactment has achieved its end.

A close cousin of enactment is projective identification, which we have touched on a bit above. Because much of the worst of the attachment trauma of neglect can begin so young, the infant brain lacks sufficient development to log explicit autobiographical memory. Rather fragments of emotion, sensation, visual "implicit" (non-story type) memory, are what are stored, and can be activated. Sometimes the only way to assemble the story is by somehow "injecting" or eliciting the feeling into another who may be more able to verbalize, (a mysterious process!) That may very well be the therapist, and again an additional reminder of how essential it is for the therapist to be exquisitely conscious and receptive to all the inner workings of themselves.

One such experience I had was with Eileen, a young woman who had minimal memory of her childhood at all. I had the suspicion that her neglect story began very early, but we had little to go on. One day in a session a powerful event occurred to help us construct her narrative. It being a session during the Pandemic, it was a remote session and I was even more focused than usual on all the subtleties inside of myself.

At a given moment in our session, Eileen turned away to reach for her shiny bright red mug of coffee and took a few sips with a purposeful expression on her face, lingering there briefly. In that moment a vivid image flashed in my mind, from a video I saw many decades ago in graduate school. Another grainy 1967 black and white, it illustrated the crucial developmental experience of the mother infant gaze, both in brain and character development. The scene I spontaneously revisited was of a narcissistic young mother and her baby of barely a couple of months.

Ideally, the infants are allowed freely to rest in a loving mutual gaze with the mother, taking periodic "breaks" by turning away when needed, to relax from the stimulation of sustained contact, only to return presently for more. This early experience results in the discovery of a rhythm of self-regulation: the comfortable pendulation and balance between arousal and recovery, sympathetic and parasympathetic brain development. With support and permission, the child begins even at this tender age, to evolve this.

The mother anxiously relished, gobbled up her baby's adoring attention, and could not tolerate even the momentary breaks in contact. When the baby attempted to turn his head away, she almost reflexively, firmly shoved it back into the gaze with her. Even when he fussed a bit, she kept his head positioned where she wanted it, all attention squarely on herself. I had to wonder, why did this pop up in my mind's eye just then? Might it be information about Eileen? Thinking about her behavior and vulnerabilities it seemed it could be. At that point, I could only take note of it and file it. But I have learned to take consider moments like that because very often they are mysterious missives from the client's unconscious to me. Not very scientific perhaps, but the psychoanalytic tradition recognizes and elaborates on these abstract phenomena. We do well to keep all channels open. This client and I were later to learn much more, that fragment by fragment fleshed out a concrete narrative of parental narcissism and neglect.

I was later to ask Eileen more about her relationship with her mother. Of course she does not remember her infancy, but she can describe their phone conversations even now. Her mother lives on the far coast, but she feels similarly stifled, unfree and as if their relationship is all about gratifying her insatiable mother. Eileen then becomes able to comprehend and feel more empathic and less ashamed for her seemingly "excessive" need for space.

Faced with self-reliance, help resistance and often extreme ambivalence from the neglect client, it may be a mystery for a while: "What are they doing here?" Or "What am I doing here?" Especially as with a client like Gail, who would often, if I began to speak (which I did not do that much with her,) would interrupt me and finish my sentence – invariably inaccurately. She thought she was having a conversation but she was "being" both of us. Or Aaron, who routinely refused to do anything I might recommend, even if it had been originally his own idea, or even if he had done it before and it really worked for him. It might be a simple somatic practice to quiet his hyper-aroused nervous system, or taking a quick walk when he had put in too many hours working at his computer, and his back felt crampy and exhausted. He categorically refused, repeatedly "shooting himself in the foot." Even though he could see that he defied his own objective, he persisted as if his life depended on it. I learned to understand these interactions as an assertion, even insistence upon existence. By doing things his own way, he had a momentary sense of having some impact, some control over *something*. And this dynamic opened a channel to many stories of his mother's not only rejection of him and anything distinct or original of his own but also her obliterating narcissism that simply dismissed whatever did not originate with herself. I had to learn not to get lost and slip into the content, or participate in an argument, but stay outside of it and work with the process, which again, provided more elements of the story. And even if he was also skeptical about looking at or remembering his childhood, in spite of himself he found it interesting and even began wondering if there were not a more positive and adaptive way to exist, that would not thwart his own objectives.

Learning the neglected client's story together may be a winding, slow trek, requiring humility, patience, versatility, creativity, and the ability to sit with the resounding message "I don't need you." It is also a powerful and momentous event for both of us, when one day they realize that they do.

## SUMMING UP AND WHAT TO DO

- Mining and assembling the narrative of a child of neglect, is a multisensory operation, requiring the therapist's patient, attentive and persistent use of their whole self, and most likely a fair amount of time.
- Narrative does matter, it is integral to having a coherent sense of self. And even if at first it does not matter to the client, it has meaning that it matters to the therapist, whether or not the client is aware of that.
- The client may come with a completely distinct agenda and presenting problem that does not include examining their childhoods. We must of course begin with what they bring. They may or may not become interested in taking it deeper eventually. We must be flexible and respectful about that.
- Modes of communication are often complex and not immediately discernible. They also may require the therapist's ability to hold unsavory or painful affects.
- The therapist must have sufficient self-knowledge and the ability to differentiate their own material from what the client is entrusting them with, or attempting to understand about themselves. Some reading about projective identification and enactment are recommended.
- Attention to nuance is required.
- Relationship therapy can be a particularly effective way of accessing the client's story, as the conflict with the partner is likely to be the most potent and direct route to story. Couples work also brings unique challenges, as "sharing a person" or scant emotional resources and sufficient attention to go around may be delicate vulnerabilities.
- Awareness of the client's body as another messenger of story is paramount, as is the availability of somatic interventions.
- Humility and the willingness to readily own and self-correct for misinterpretations and missteps are particularly meaningful and necessary.

## BIBLIOGRAPHY

Bell, David. "Projective Identification." In *Kleinian Theory: A Contemporary Perspective*, edited by Catalina Bronstein, 125–147. London: Whurr, 2001.

Coates, Ta-Nehisi. *The Water Dancer*. New York: One World, 2019.

Lanius, Ruth A., Braeden A. Terpou, and Margaret C. McKinnon. "The Sense of Self in the Aftermath of Trauma: Lessons from the Default Mode Network in Posttraumatic Stress Disorder." *European Journal of Psychotraumatology* 11, no. 1 (October 2020). https://doi.org/10.1080/2 0008198.2020.1807703.

Lanius, Ruth A., Peter C. Williamson, Maria Densmore, Kristine Boksman, R. W. Neufeld, Joseph S. Gati, and Ravi S. Menon. "The Nature of Traumatic Memories: A 4-T fMRI Functional Connectivity Analysis." *American Journal of Psychiatry* 161, no. 1 (January 2004): 36–44. https://doi.org/10.1176/appi.ajp.161.1.36.

Levine, Peter A. *In an Unspoken Voice: How the Body Releases Trauma and Restores Goodness*. Berkeley, California: North Atlantic Books, 2010.

Van der Kolk, Bessel A. "Trauma and Memory." *Psychiatry and Clinical Neurosciences* 52, no. S1 (September 1998): S52–S64. https://doi.org/10.1046/j.1440-1819.1998.0520s5S97.x.

Van der Kolk, Bessel A. *The Body Keeps the Score: Brain, Mind, and Body in the Healing of Trauma*. New York: Penguin Books, 2014.

Van der Kolk, Bessel A., and Onno van der Hart. "Pierre Janet and the Breakdown of Adaptation in Psychological Trauma." *American Journal of Psychiatry* 146, no. 12 (December 1989): 1530–40. https://doi.org/10.1176/ajp.146.12.1530.

# Chapter 5

# Emotion: Teaching a Foreign Language

For those of us whose world has always been painted with a wide spectrum of emotion, replete with shading and nuance, it is difficult to imagine living without them. Although at times in my life, I have felt cursed by feeling "too much," I wholeheartedly value the depth and range of perception and experience emotional tone and variety add to my life. Additionally, emotion is not a "luxury" or a superfluous function, but has an essential evolutionary and survival function. A life of muted or absent emotion is not only flat but also lacking vital perceptual information. In this chapter, we will explore the impoverished emotional landscape of the child of neglect. Why emotions matter; what are the consequences and sequelae both from inside and outside the client, of minimal emotion? How do emotion and its absence interplay with story and memory? And most importantly, how do we teach or facilitate accessing, identifying or naming, experiencing and expressing emotion? Or even before that, how might we "sell" them to individuals who may have made a lifelong practice and even priority of meticulously avoiding them?

## WHY EMOTIONS MATTER

Emotion has vital significance to survival, and registers danger and threat in the most primitive regions of the reptilian brain well before we can even feel it, and compels immediate action to achieve safety. Frank Corrigan has written elegantly about this process and has devised a treatment protocol to both bring these initial warning signals to awareness, and process the historical "residue" which may persist in the body or unconscious. Well beyond acute and immediate danger that would require quick and urgent action, like yanking a child out of oncoming traffic, emotion registers information from the external and internal world that merits attention, and perhaps sooner than cognition might. An example of the external world might be, the appearance of a strange man in a young child's close vicinity. An example of information from the internal world, or the world inside the body, Rachel after systematically starving herself over long periods in her life, could not readily feel the sensations of hunger anymore. But later in recovery, an intrusion of quiet fear might poke through from the inside if she felt dizziness or stomach rumblings, that she was not eating enough that day.

We are all familiar with the fight flight response, survival strategies also activated by fear. Less familiar might be the freeze response for the cases when physical self-defense or escape are impossible. Freeze or collapse is a last line of defense, as Peter Levine demonstrates artfully with vignettes from the animal world. An animal who is cornered, with no other options, may "feign death" or "play possum" in the hope that the predator thinking it is dead, will lose interest, or to numb against the inescapable pain of being eaten. This is often the case with our developmental trauma clients, and may help explain the effective and perhaps even habitual numbing we might often see in neglect clients. Practiced at this "management" of the dilemma, it may have become a default state.

Emotion also informs us about the intentions of the others. Granted the child of neglect may misread emotional cues. Ideally, however, emotion as a way to register the intent of others, is part of nature's design. With luck, they may if read accurately, elicit empathy and connection, also essential for humans. After all, we are pack animals and inherently interdependent. Pat Love reminds us that altruism evokes a dopamine surge, a blast of pleasure, re-enforcing an adaptive behavior supporting survival of the interdependent group. And anecdotally I discovered first in myself in my early practice of neurofeedback, that the opposite of joy may not be sorrow, but at least in my case, fear. The calmer I became the happier I felt. My joy informed me that I was emerging from fear. Clearly there are many good reasons why emotions are necessary and worth it, although the child of neglect, having experienced a poverty of the good ones, may not agree, and misses out on a wealth and depth of experience of self and other.

## HOW DOES EMOTIONAL FLUENCY BEGIN?

John Gottman the marriage researcher developed an elegant and simple approach called "Emotionally Coached Parenting" which details how one teaches emotional intelligence to young children. It is illuminating and explicit and I find it to be of use at any age. (I might recommend it to couples, especially couples where one or both are a child of neglect.) Essentially, a child learns to recognize what they are feeling, through having it reflected in the caregiver's eyes.

If an infant looks up into the eyes of the caregiver, and sees a reflection of themselves, they will first of all feel connected, which will later translate to a sense of value, "I matter," If they feel scared or in pain, and they see that feeling reflected back in the parent's eyes or expression, and the parent responds by accurately meeting the need, the child not only feels gratified and met, and therefore safe, but also begins to become familiar with the emotion, understand it in relation to the need expressed. If the parent additionally combines language with the experience, the child begins to develop a file, developed where the need, the feeling experience, the response and even eventually the name of the feeling are housed increasing integrated, together. A growing lexicon of emotion is learned. This is obviously not conscious for a long time. But little circuits are growing and that is what we want the client to understand.

I might readily say to a client, "If I look up into your eyes and I see a reflection of me, a smiling and warm reflection of me as if I am a source of pleasure and joy, I will feel pleasure and joy, and calm. If I am scared and I look up into your eyes, and see a reflection of my fear, and you say and do something comforting, I will feel not only comforted, but seen, understood, and attended to, again valued and connected. And I learn about the emotion, the need, and the response to the need."

Such an intervention may be moving to a client, especially if they are parents themselves, or have a beloved pet whom they adoringly attend to in this way. It may bring tears, even if the client does not know why. It may bring bits of story, such as when Ralph noted matter-of-factly "I was in an incubator for the first 20 days of my life ..." a significant, and illuminating "detail that I had not heard about him before."

Emotion may bring  fragments of memory. For example, when Wendy recalled, "I remember when I had my tonsils out when I was two. I woke up in that room and it was dark. I was terrified. I was so cold and my throat hurt, and there was nobody there. And they had promised me that when I got my tonsils out, I would get ice cream. Where was the ice cream? I cried and cried, but nobody seemed to hear, and nobody came. All I know is that after that I avoided hospitals at all costs, and I didn't really know why."

Our mirroring function, which continues to be my redundant (and tiresome?) refrain, seeks to repair this missing essential experience. Perhaps slowing down the recounting of the memory fragment, will bring a flash of the fear, an image of the darkroom, a momentary blast of cold, a pain in the throat. Whatever comes, we focus on and ask the client to hold, preferably as much as possible to still the various sensory components together. We stay empathically present with all of that, and attempt to hold them there as long as they can tolerate it. Somatic therapy pioneer Al Pesso might add "If I were there then, I would have ..." supplying the missing responsive caretaking behavior. If there is a partner present to say this, even better. This helps to both integrate the memory, make sense out of it, educate about emotion, and re-enforce the experience of an empathic other. The calming impact as well as insight gained from this intervention, may help us in our "case" about why emotion has any value at all. Additionally, if we are treating the child of neglect in couples therapy, the partner may have been longing for more moments of emotion breaking through, and respond with love, admiration and additional comfort for the neglected child.

## EMOTION AND THE BRAIN

For a more neuroscience-based view, which some clients (but certainly not all) find reassuring, Allan Schore's work, as referenced in Chapter 1, explicitly emphasizes that the infant brain grows and develops through the resonance, right hemisphere to right hemisphere, of the infant brain to the caregiver's brain. At least that is how it is supposed to be. The right hemisphere is the home of much emotional function, and because the circuitry of emotion develops much earlier than the more advanced circuitry of cognition, emotion will be much of the language of this early resonance.

In addition to the essential emotional skills and capabilities we have already named, (identifying, feeling, naming and expressing them) Schore spotlights the vital function of *self-regulation,* that the child eventually, it is hoped, learns through the resonance. By regulation we mean from the experience of being calmed and soothed, thereby brought back to a comfortable homeostatic baseline by the attentive caregiver, the child ultimately becomes able to do that for themselves. They learn to calm themselves down.

And what if this resonance is unreliable, deficient, inaccurate, frightening or simply absent? Essential developmental tasks may fail to advance. If this *self-regulation* is not learned, and the child lacks training in how to return to baseline, after becoming scared, confused, frustrated or in some way agitated or "hyper-aroused," they can get stuck there, unable to recover and get back to calm, which makes emotion a dicey undertaking. It makes sense that such a child would learn to clamp down against their emotions. Perhaps then, this suggests that the emotional (or non-emotional as it were) world of neglect goes beyond parental failures of empathy and understanding. The child is left alone, perhaps under siege, in the confusing and often stormy universe of emotion.

Stan learned to "walk on eggshells" or judiciously avoid interactions with Cora that would set him or them off. Being painfully unable to calm down after getting upset, the aftermath of an episode might last for a week or more. He lived in dread of the next one. Learning to calm himself down, some of which of course involved experiencing repair from relationship rupture, was sadly missing from his attachment history. Acquiring those capacities greatly reduced his baseline fear and agitation level, which in spite of himself he found made the therapy worthwhile.

Infants are particularly sensitive and hyper-attuned to the response and lack or absence of response of the caregiver, right from the start, and for quite some time thereafter. Infant psychiatrist Ed Tronick devised an exquisitely illustrative study called the "Still Face" that powerfully portrays this. In his experiment, a securely attached infant is happily playing with his mother, who also appears to be delightedly enjoying herself. At a designated point, she is instructed to shift to a blank or expressionless "still face" – not angry and not

overtly intimidating, simply expressionless, for approximately 2 minutes. The baby first baffled, tries to discover what has happened.
Where did she go? He then tries desperately to bring her back, by
being cute attempting to continue the play. He tries tugging at her,
much like my little dog who keeps pawing at me to continue petting
her, when I am trying to type which requires both of my hands. In
much less than the two minutes, the "Still Face" child is first fussing
and then full-on wailing. And this is a still and expressionless face,
not an angry face or a tearful or depressed face, or a frightened face
or a frightening or a missing face, but a neutral one. Even that has a
catastrophic impact. Imagine the experience of that child when this
continues for more than two minutes; there is no one there, or the
caregiver is threatening, sad, rageful or somehow out of control.

The Still Face videos are readily and freely accessible, and well
worth watching. Often describing the experiment to a client has
quite an effect, and may elicit thoughtful recall about where the
mother was, or what was going on in her life, when the client was an
infant, valuable not only with respect to emotion but also from an
elaboration of narrative standpoint as well. It may alternatively elicit
remembered stories from when they were older, like Suzie's memory of looking up at her mother's bereft and terrified face, after
another loud argument with her father that resulted in his storming
out of the house and being gone for days.

Many of our neglected clients are hugely intelligent, in a way I
used to find almost intimidating, especially when there are fancy
titles and fancy schools involved. Until I met Nick, a surgeon who
had not only studied and trained at a top university but additionally
had a PhD from another one. Discovering that poor Nick just needed
a mom, like everyone else, was like encountering Miss Wiesjahn in
the grocery store. As intelligent as these clients are, they may be
equally void of emotional intelligence. Sometimes great intelligence
is even an obstacle, as they reflexively default to what they may ency-
clopedically know. Pointing this out, "Sometimes extraordinarily
smart people have a harder time with emotion!" which contains
both a compliment, while it names and perhaps also makes sense of
this weakness, may be effective. Or the weakness, or disability may
not occur to them, unless someone like a partner complains of it,
placing it on the radar, and even then, they may discount it. My
experience has been, although many might initially prefer to die
rather than enter a feeling world, once they become more fluent, or

experience a benefit, their rejection or at the very least avoidance of emotion softens or opens, and they experience great relief.

I must add, that emotion and its expression are still viewed as a weakness in men, and a flaw in women. Many women are still excluded from key authoritative roles with such a "rationale." Many of our male clients remember being shamed or ridiculed for expressions of emotion or God forbid, tears. Jim remembers when he was four and his sister precipitously died, of mysterious and incomprehensible causes. No one bothered to talk to him, or to consider, let alone address his distress, or to help him in anyway comprehend what had happened. Shocked and confused, he collapsed into overwhelmed tears. His father was quick to ceremoniously and publicly scold him, loudly reprimanding him to "Be a man!" Jim learned that emotion, and most of all tears, were to be hidden at the very least, if not banished entirely. Of course, his recourse to early substance abuse and subsequent addiction "helped" with that, and these messages to boys and girls, are sadly still most alive and "well" in our culture.


## THE WORK WITH EMOTION

As noted, it may be a hard sell that emotion even has value in its own right. Many of our neglected clients have gotten by more comfortably in life, or protected themselves by skillfully keeping emotion at bay. They may be aware that they do not care to rock that boat, thanks. They may or may not be aware that they dislike emotion, they may find emotions unwieldy, messy and disorderly, "illogical" a diversion, distraction or "waste of time." Especially fear and sadness are not only unpleasant but also inconvenient, so what is the point of indulging such unpleasantness?

They probably are not aware of how much the emotions (that they may not even realize that they have), influence their thinking and decision making. Rachel in the height of her anorexia was sent one time to a psychiatrist whom she found scarily and nauseatingly lascivious, as well as inattentive; and way too quick to want to just "slap her on meds." She was immediately aware that she was *never* going back to him, but not quite sure why, nor why she never again rode her bike down the street where his office was, in all the remaining years that she continued to live in her hometown.

It may be a while before we are able to break it to our clients, that with or without their notice, they are filled with feelings. And those feelings do show themselves. When Rachel volunteered the story about her doctor, and I was able to slow her down enough to get detail, there were faint glimmers of feeling in her eyes. Partly it was rather dazzling and unfamiliar that anyone was curious about her world. She had never talked about what it was like to be severely anorexic in the early 1960s. No one knew anything then, so she readily accepted her parents' interpretation that she was "just bad!" and creating unnecessary stress for them. Entombed in shame, it had been hidden and locked away for years.

A word we will hear often is what I think of as the catch-all umbrella term "overwhelmed," which is vague and imprecise, and clearly connotes too much of something. But I will want to know too much of what? I think of it as overstimulated, but again, if they are able to slow it down and be descriptive, it helps me to get a picture or a feel for their interior or their past, and it helps them to practice or learn to speak about their feeling of whatever kind. Little glimmers of emotion may poke through, and if we name that, we may or may not elicit more. In Rachel's case, she had always wished someone might want to know, and listen, without fully realizing that. When I said, "You look so sad." She said, "I am just overwhelmed." I was uncertain if she was overstimulated by the memory, or by the experience of someone wanting to know, or even just remembering what little she could about those desperate and lonely years. What I will attempt to do is find out more about what it is like, the "phenomenology" of overwhelm, or what it is like from every angle. They may or may not have the interest, the patience or the words for it. But they may in fact find it a rewarding journey of discovery.

I have observed that word "anxious," often connotes the suppression of emotion. It takes a lot of energy to keep emotions under the lid, so to speak, and that can be agitating at best. It is often hard to sell that "befriending" or at least allowing them is inherently calming. Admittedly, I am a stickler for words, how differently different clients may use the same word. I will always at least attempt to find out, what that word "means to you" which they might welcome or find annoying, or both. I might need to offer a menu, does it mean "flooded with too much feeling at once?" "Or pitched into a pit of numbness?" "Is it scary?" Whatever I can think of and what I might hear is "that feeling makes me want to vomit, and sometimes I do." The gentle probing may also be a vehicle for fine tuning their own emotional self-perception, and the likelihood of being more accurately known and understood.

A note of caution, sometimes (but not only) if for example, the neglect is laced or layered with overt trauma, tapping into the defense too soon or too quickly may unleash the very flood of "overwhelm" in itself. Lisa was one such, and in an early session before I knew her well, I inquired too much too soon, or at the very least I failed to stop or slow her down enough. She felt "too much," "overdisclosed" and did not get out of bed for a week. She was afraid to return to therapy.

The mirroring function *never* upstages the mandate to keep the client safe. And precision and slow thoughtful inquiry, utilizing available memory fragments, carefully dosed and paced, and with close attention for any breakthrough indication or emotion, are important ways that we work. And sometimes, we will learn, that the important breakthrough glimmer happened outside the session, when they were safely and customarily alone. They may tell us about it, and we may be able to take them back to it, perhaps taking it further or deeper.

## EMOTION AND THE BODY

From our keenly focused attention, we must watch for the cues that there may be emotion, hidden from view, that we may begin to acknowledge and name. A rich resource, of course, is the client's body. Corrigan reminds us that the Periaqueductal Gray, which is where we first register that initial "yank-the-toddler out of oncoming traffic" fear response, the "orienting response" has rich connections to the body. The treatment protocol he has created, "Deep Brain Re-orienting" (DBR) targets the manifest body sensations where it will be first discernible, before the emotion comes to awareness. These are located in the back of the neck, and many of our neglect clients report pain, stiffness aching or stuck-ness in the neck and back. Corrigan's protocol, working from both somatic and neuroscience expertise, is elegant, simple, (and far from easy) and powerfully effective. It heightens awareness of both body sensation and emotion. And if our neglect client has the patience, it can be administered remotely, a perk during this protracted global Pandemic. It also means that clients could be referred to Frank, who is in Scotland, or someone he has trained who might be most anywhere in the world. I have not studied it yet, but it is the next modality on my list. Suffice it to say here, the body is a gold mine of information, which may or may not be accessible to the child of neglect. But we certainly want to at least, gently lower the spade, which may not be easy at all. But it might.

And how do we know that there is emotion lurking? We must be scrupulously attentive for not only emotional but also somatic cues or clues. Lorraine had disabling and seemingly intractable cycling headaches that were impossible to ignore. They seemed impervious to the range of headache medications. She was not aware of an emotion they might be trying to express. But when we began to use a neurofeedback migraine protocol, the emotion began to surface as profound and pervasive anger. The headaches began to slowly respond to the treatment, but the availability of the anger, enabled us to process that, which made for a dramatic shift in the treatment progress that would have never been possible with talk alone. Bessel van der Kolk's now ubiquitous, The Body Keeps the Score is certainly applicable to developmental trauma and neglect. It details a wide range of somatic approaches. I studied and became certified in almost all of them over the years, but I continue to return to and favor neurofeedback (although it was temporarily disrupted by the Pandemic), which I will say more about in Chapter 10. Along with van der Kolk's book, I highly recommend, Sebern Fisher's book about neurofeedback in the treatment of developmental trauma, to the interested reader.

Being trained and skilled at some somatic treatment approach(es) or at the very least having known and trusted referrals for such, is essential for accessing often elusive emotion in children of neglect. It is always preferable to administer the somatic practice, whatever it is, oneself, when humanly possible. My father used to say that "reading poetry in translation, is like kissing a bride through a veil." I feel similarly about splitting the treatment, and diluting the challenge of dependency/transference on a caregiver in this way. And it is also impractical, as too much information can be virtually impossible to exchange and share adequately between providers.

In talk therapy, be attuned to any change in pace of speech, halting or quickening. A change in tone, tension, movement, posture, hands or jaw tightening, gaze or voice; and of course, the eyes, which are the window where we can most readily see the shadow of sorrow and pain if it is anywhere near. Edward, although he was exquisitely vigilant to anger in others, rarely registered his own. I learned to recognize a subtle guttural lowering of his voice, as a clue that he was himself angry, (and sometimes angry with me). Lorraine might suddenly and subtly begin to smile during the neurofeedback, which I might and inquire about later.

I attempt to track myself carefully, *listening to whatever the narrative at this stage may evoke: perhaps an emotional response or image in me* that may seem *noteworthy* enough to merit exploration. (There is virtually always a song in my head, and I have learned to give them notice as well!) When Rhonda's company laid off a quarter of the workforce during the Corona Virus Pandemic, she was spared, and able to maintain her much needed income. Racked with survivor guilt and self-doubt, she was quick to explain that she remained employed "*only*" because she was Black.

She stated matter-of-factly, "I happen to *know* that a number of my white co-workers who did lose their jobs, were much better performers, more ambitious and more competent than I am. They just kept me because in these times it looks good to have racial diversity. *It is just plain 'good optics.'*" It was a ready conclusion; a default given that her lifelong explanation to herself for being ignored and forgotten, was that she was not "good enough" not enough, or simply could not compete. If the assumption was always "I am worthless" such a conclusion about staying employed made sense.

Early in the therapy it may be difficult or simply untimely to attempt to evoke childhood connections, it may sound dismissive to them, or as if we are not listening or "getting" what they are saying *now,* or that what they are saying is important in real time, (which it also is). If that is the case, we "file" it. And we may be able to refer back to the layoffs at some later time. In our case, Rhonda being impressively intelligent and thoughtful, it was difficult for me to believe that she was as incapable and unworthy as she described. The gnawing inside myself emboldened me enough to inquire further. I was able to say "How do you know?" And when her response was tepid and unconvincing, I could ask her, "Is that a familiar feeling or belief, 'I am not good enough'?"

Rhonda was not able or interested in making those connections yet, it was only several weeks later when she brought in photos (also an effective stimulus when available), of her large family. In some she was tiny, and very young, not much more than a toddler. In others she was older. In all of them she looked heartbreakingly sad and far away. She herself could see that, and memory fragments floated gradually to the surface. She herself began to recall thoughts that would conjure first the idea, and then the emotional memory of loneliness, feeling inadequate, unloved and even angry.

As noted, clients who are themselves parents, often appear to be quite good ones, capable of exquisite attunement and empathy. Of course, what we have to go on is their report, but nonetheless, we may intuit something. Randy noticed that as his little daughter became increasingly verbal, she was also asking Randy many questions about how the world worked, the perennial "why, Daddy?" about many things. Randy when first telling me about this, got an unfamiliar, distant (to me) look in his eyes. Tracking that we tapped into deep longings and sadness, a wish he could now faintly remember, longing for a reliable other whom he could ask. "I had to be re-inventing the wheel endlessly."

I then witnessed the first appearance in our therapy, of Randy's copious tears. Later if Randy hit a wall, blocking access to his emotion about something, be it from childhood or present time, I might ask, "What do you think that would be like for Susie?" Or "what would you feel if that happened to her?" invariably, the path would open to his previously "lost" feeling.


## NOT METAPHOR

I like to say, "metaphor is great for poetry, but not for communication in relationship." They may be aesthetically pleasing but they are obfuscating. And they divert the client away from emotion. I will hear them out, and possibly file their image for some later reference, and then attempt to access emotion. Metaphor generally takes them to cognition. I attempt to teach them to go straight for a feeling word, which is much more likely to connect them with the feeling in question, itself. Again, a menu of options, may be helpful. If we hit on it, it is likely to be connecting, both of the client with themselves, and also perhaps with me. Similarly, it is more direct (much less familiar) and much more potent, to use the first person singular, i.e. "I feel," rather than "*it* feels like …" details of communication that can be hugely significant in both emotional experience, and also eliciting accurate empathy.

As noted, other directedness and the experience of being invisible or nonexistent, may have cemented the habit of answering the question of how they feel, with their perception of the feeling state of the other, whomever that might be. "I felt like she was fed up with me," keeping them at a "safe" distance from their own experience, where the more accurate "I was panicked that she was going to disappear again" would have taken us more directly to the material that would make a difference. "In their own yard," is where the healing is bringing them back to their *own* experience is a reminder not only that their feelings have merit and value to themselves but even to the listener, in this case me; but also more fundamentally that they do *exist.*

Later in the therapy, the client may become blessedly able to connect the emotional dots themselves, contacting the previously foreign or distant emotional experience. Jackie doggedly hanging in through the challenges of COVID 19, found herself wearing down at about the five-month mark. She had already realized that the government's response, or rather lack thereof, to the dire circumstances, reminded her too much of her mother's global obliviousness to her throughout her childhood, including when circumstances were threatening and uncertain, and similarly dire. Although we were meeting regularly via video, she missed our twice weekly neurofeedback (more about this in Chapter 10) sessions. She had been proud and happy about how the neurofeedback results had lasted, but she was beginning to worry that perhaps they were fading.

In one of our sessions, she acknowledged, "I was feeling kind of dark, and could not seem to shake it." She was worried by self-disparaging thoughts and preoccupations about her body and her weight. She now knew without question, that those thoughts and feelings, were not the "real" issue, and she came to interpret them to be a communication that she was "out of balance," and needed to decipher that. Still at least a part of her was afraid she would lapse into the deadly "comfort-eating" that had both sustained and plagued her through childhood and beyond. She *really* did not want that!

Jackie was always hesitant to call a friend when she felt low. She now had a small number of real friends, but still and most certainly (and typical among children of neglect), did not want to need or impose. But now for the first time under such circumstances, she called her friend Andrea. They were able to share their frustrations about politics, and then talk about some of the craft and gardening ideas that they enjoyed and shared. They got together for a COVID safe visit out in Andrea's yard, and spent the afternoon.

"When I got home, I felt better! And much less 'hungry!'" Jackie exclaimed apparently surprised by the discovery. "I need more connection!" It was actually radical for her. "Isolation is boring! Booooring!" and she dipped into sorrowful recollection about the endless isolation, boredom, loneliness, self-hatred and self-destructive eating, that were the story of her childhood. Yes, the work of emotion is an essential task of our work with these clients.

It behooves the therapist to assemble a fluent vocabulary of feeling words. I used to go online and look for the cute charts with lists of emotions, often illustrated with line drawing emoji-like faces, that I could hand out as a reference and practice guide. There are many good ones. I don't do that so much anymore. If you are not an "emotion hound" like me, and I unapologetically tell my clients I am, I recommend at the very least to develop a familiarity, facility and a sizeable glossary. Like color, flavor, humor and variety, emotion may *seem* non-essential to them. All of these are certainly essential to me and they temper the blandness, redundancy or what may be seemingly unending existential distress about the state of the world, in addition to enhancing life with dimension, texture and aliveness. Emotion is in a different category, however. Beside its other survival functions, it is vital for self and other knowledge and connection, which also are what makes existence and life worthwhile.

## SUMMING UP AND WHAT TO DO

- Emotion is essential for a variety of reasons. It has vital survival functions of signaling danger and threat to incite appropriate and necessary action. It facilitates and cements attachment and empathic connection, which we as interdependent and pack animals, require. Although the neglect experience trains the client against acknowledging it or even feeling it. Emotion is not a luxury, and living without it may explain feeling deadened, bored and empty.

- Ideally emotional intelligence and emotional fluency are learned in earliest childhood, through the attachment experience of infant with primary caregiver. The resonance between them, right hemisphere to right hemisphere, begin to develop its circuitry, concurrent with attachment. Because right hemisphere, emotional function develops well in advance of the left more cognitive hemisphere, emotion will be a first language. When as with neglect, this early resonance is insufficient or lacking, that language is not learned, or its learning is derailed or somehow disturbed, or even virtually non-existent. A vital task of therapy is to attempt to replicate the emotional learning process, which may initially be counter-intuitive or undesirable to the client, at least at first.

- Various forms of dysregulation result from the neglected child's missing attachment experiences. Most significantly the child, without sufficient comfort and mirroring, lacks the experience of returning to baseline, when attachment has been ruptured, or when over-stimulated in some unpleasant or threatening way. They are left alone and defenscless, thrown on their own underdeveloped resources to get back to homeostasis, which is clearly too much for an infant or small child. The child then creates defenses and strategies to compensate and cope.

- For each particular client, we must find the methodologies most effective for awakening and re-instating emotion. Many are nonverbal as the verbal left hemisphere has historically always dominated and predominated the child of neglect's behavior and function.

- The body is a rich mine and potentially minefield if we are not careful, of emotional communication and access. Learning to translate communication from the body is key.

- Of course talk therapy will be at least one component of this work. But only one among others.

## BIBLIOGRAPHY

Corrigan, Frank M., and Alastair M. Hull. "Recognition of the Neurobiological Insults Imposed by Complex Trauma and the Implications for Psychotherapeutic Interventions." *BJPsych Bulletin* 39, no. 2 (April 2015): 79–86. https://doi.org/10.1192/pb.bp.114.047134.
Fisher, Sebern F. *Neurofeedback in the Treatment of Developmental Trauma: Calming the Fear-Driven Brain.* New York: W. W. Norton, 2014.

Gottman, John, and Joan Declaire. *Raising an Emotionally Intelligent Child: The Heart of Parenting*. New York: Fireside, 1998.

Ham, Jacob, and Ed Tronick. "Infant Resilience to the Stress of the Still-Face: Infant and Maternal Psychophysiology Are Related." *Annals of the New York Academy of Sciences* 1094, no. 1 (December 2006): 297–302. https://doi.org/10.1196/annals.1376.038.

Levine, Peter A. *In an Unspoken Voice: How the Body Releases Trauma and Restores Goodness*. Berkeley, California: North Atlantic Books, 2010.

Love, Patricia, and Steven Stosny. *How to Improve Your Marriage Without Talking about It*. New York: Broadway Books, 2007.

Panksepp, Jaak. *Affective Neuroscience: The Foundations of Human and Animal Emotions*. Series in Affective Science. New York: Oxford University Press, 1998.

Pesso, Albert. "Pesso Boyden System Psychomotor." In *The Illustrated Encyclopedia of Body-Mind Disciplines*, edited by Nancy Allison, 411–415. New York: Rosen Publishing Group, 1999.

Schore, Allan N. *Affect Regulation and the Origin of the Self: The Neurobiology of Emotional Development*. New York: Routledge, 2016. First published 1994 by Lawrence Erlbaum Associates (Hillsdale, New Jersey).

Schwarz, Lisa, Frank Corrigan, Alastair M. Hull, and Rajiv Raju. *The Comprehensive Resource Model: Effective Therapeutic Techniques for the Healing of Complex Trauma*. Explorations in Mental Health. New York: Routledge, 2017.

Sonne, Don M., and Gash. "Psychopathy to Altruism: Neurobiology of the Selfish–Selfless Spectrum." *Frontiers in Psychology* 9, no. 575 (April 2018). https://doi.org/10.3389/fpsyg.2018.00575.

Twomey, Steve. "Phineas Gage: Neuroscience's Most Famous Patient." *Smithsonian*, January 2010. https://www.smithsonianmag.com/history/phineas-gage-neurosciences-most-famous-patient-11390067/.

Van der Kolk, Bessel A. *The Body Keeps the Score: Brain, Mind, and Body in the Healing of Trauma*. New York: Penguin Books, 2014.

# Chapter 6

# Sexuality: Unraveling the Conundrum of Need

Neglect first came to my awareness in a largely sexual context. That sexual trauma often engenders sexual difficulties, psychological, somatic and even medical, is not news. Many of my first women survivor clients were plagued by every sort of sexual symptom and difficulty, not least of them being partners' "demands" that they felt ill-equipped, paralyzed, terrified or simply unwilling to gratify. They felt unsupported, not understood, henpecked and increasingly unhappy with their partners. Both partners felt already massively stressed by the seemingly endless trauma healing process, which was both financially and "metabolically" expensive.

Back then we had much less research, knowledge about trauma in general, and sill less about trauma and sex. When in 2017, I was asked to do a formal literature review on the subject I was distressed but not surprised by how little research and data were as yet available at the interface. Some good clinical work is at last happening in many places, and I can attest to healing and growth in this area in my own work, however, a solid evidence base is still needed. Similarly, back then, we had little specialized methodology to move things along.

Life was grim for those couples and families, and as I got to know them, I learned that many had not had sex with their spouses in years. I remember when I met my first couple who had not had sex in 10 years. The male partner was then 40. It was unimaginable to a child of the Free Love Generation like me. And interestingly infidelity rarely intruded, at least with live partners. I found myself to be similarly ill-equipped, to be helpful, and promptly began my training and later certification in sex therapy. Thankfully I have learned much since those long past days.

Beyond my deep attachment focus, I have always had a special interest in sexuality, and from the start of my career, was somatically oriented, and profoundly interested in the body, and the mind-body interplay. Sex brings together, body, mind and relationship, in ways that are complex, challenging and to me, fascinating. Studying the workings of the brain adds yet another dimension, as do the social, political and moral taboos surrounding sex. All this is the lens through which we will examine neglect in this chapter.

A unique aspect of sexuality, is the simultaneous interaction between arousal, or excitement, and calm; stimulation and ease; sympathetic and parasympathetic. As Harville Hendrix pointed out in one of his first books for couples, "safety and passion ..." If partners do not feel safe, there will be no passion, and effectively no sex. Even animals in the wild know this, and will stop what they are doing immediately if there is a predator in the vicinity. An extreme of a unique and delicate self-regulation is required to keep these seemingly contradictory flows of energy in balance. In the child of neglect, challenges of relationship, self-regulation and need, converge, in the larger context of a complex sociopolitical, moral world.

An additional twist for me has been that in my thirty-five-plus years of passionately inhabiting both the trauma and sexuality fields, there has been distressingly little cross-pollination between them. I have felt like the child of distant, estranged parents, not necessarily antagonistic, but too busy and preoccupied to have any interest in the other. Or so it seemed to me. I made my best effort at building the bridge myself, but it took years to make headway with that. Now that the ACE Study has become mainstream common fare, and PTSD is part of the public lexicon, there is a new awareness and concern with being "trauma-informed." In the last couple of years, the sex therapy field has taken steps to educate sex therapists about trauma. The trauma field less so, but I don't give up. All this is to say, that the child of neglect has been long ignored, and the complex sexuality that might come with neglect, to be sure.

In light of what we are coming to understand about the psychological, relational, emotional and brain/bodily dynamics of neglect, we will visit a small sampler of sexual expressions of dysregulation; examine them against a baseline of what regulated sexual health is; briefly visit what I have come to view as a more generalized public health matter surrounding sex, what that means for the child of neglect; and in the quest for healing solutions, consider what therapists can do.

I do want to acknowledge, that the examples I have offered, have been primarily heterosexual. Although I have worked with and continue to enjoy working with numerous individuals of all orientations, I have surmised that same sex couples and individuals are not inclined to seek *sexual* therapy/help from an old straight lady like me.

## THE CONUNDRUM OF NEED

For the child of neglect, whose default is self-reliance, sexuality presents a dilemma. Although it is possible to "do it all oneself," with sex it is simply not the same. Masturbation is effective in some ways, but hardly a substitute for sex with another person. This then, presents the conundrum with which our neglect survivors are faced. If relatedness is foreign, "uncomfortable" or downright dangerous that will surely show itself in the sexual realm. Many, survivors of neglect, however unconsciously, pair up with someone unavailable sexually, and re-enact the experience of being repulsive and "untouchable" by the mother. Others avoid the tangle presented by need, with a whirling tornado like flight from one partner to another, in some version of compulsive or impulsive sexual activity. Some people their sex lives with sex workers or live sex performances, an intimacy that is more in fantasy or in some way internal, that reflects their familiar or known "comfort" level with proximity and love. Some inhabit a sex life consisting of inanimate partners, via porn or movies. Some spend their lives in a constant state of gnawing "skin hunger," and longing. Perhaps they are lonely, some are not. I have had some clients who had been single for years and decades, and it was OK. Jackie, now in her late fifties, had not dated since her undergrad days. She honestly did not miss it. In this chapter, we will visit but a handful of expressions of what I view as the sexuality of neglect, all of which is anecdotal and hypothetical, however useful and effective it has proven to be for me. Nonetheless this is a large, complex and un-studied view.

## REPLICATING EARLY NEGLECT IN
## THERAPY, AND EVERYWHERE

In the early days of my work, in keeping with the larger context, there was of course a sad poverty of literature about trauma and sex. To be precise, I was able to find just one book, a self-help book on the subject of sexual healing for these individuals and couples. Wendy Malz's *The Sexual Healing Journey*, which first appeared in 1991. That one lonely volume was practical and hands-on, about things couples might try, and do, however, the heart of its message was that the partner of the designated traumatized, in this case the sexually violated client, needed to be patient and supportive, beyond saintly, a little therapist-like. In effect, they were to "disappear" or disavow their own pain and discomfort; continue to endure, wait and figure out how to manage their own physical and emotional desire and frustration about lack of sex. By the time I met these couples, that was understandably wearing thin for these men, and for many that wildly understates it.

Meanwhile, the designated trauma survivor felt increasingly guilty, pressured and retraumatized and certainly not more desirous; while the partner somehow tolerated sexless, often completely touchless "monogamy" and often for years. They both felt terribly stymied and often desperate. And it certainly did not help that no one seemed to be talking with them about sex, rather the subject seemed to be sorely neglected, or avoided. In my graduate school days, the only human sexuality requirement for graduation and licensure, was one "quickie" four-hour workshop.

Many couples I saw who had seen couples' therapists before, sometimes for a significant amount of time, had never been asked about their sexual relationship. Doctors and psychiatrists did not seem to talk about it, whether in the context of pregnancy, side effects of the then new and much touted and prescribed SSRI medications; the potential impact on sexuality of breast cancer or prostate surgery, to name just a few. Couples seemed to conclude, that talking about sex was forbidden. Or they were just already "supposed to know" which explained everyone's silence on the subject. Of course in the case of sexual abuse in the family, any mention of sex was likely to be shrouded in secrecy and shame.

The survivor of sexual trauma was the designated "problem child" while the partner was essentially sidelined, overlooked, taken for granted, in effect neglected. When my thinking coagulated around what came to be my understanding of neglect, it began to make sense to me how a childhood of neglect, could prepare and train a person for a parched desert of waiting, feeling rejected, unwanted, repelled and ashamed. This was the subject of my first book.

## REJECTION OF THE BODY

During this era, I met Ryan and Louise. Louise had a wrenching history of sexual and physical trauma, first inside her family of origin, and then outside. She was not shy about saying, that if she never had sex again for the rest of her life, that would be just fine by her. Her hideous experiences could easily monopolize and take up all the space of our therapy, if I allowed it to. Ryan, a thoughtful young man of few words, felt differently. He, like Louise, was in his middle thirties when I met them. It took some coaxing to learn about his childhood.

Ryan, a talented, even successful artist, was the elder of two children, with a self-centered and absent mother. At times she seemed depressed, at other times she drank, still other times, Ryan could not figure out why she was so distant and rejecting of him for as long as he could remember. He really could not figure her out in general. Now as she got older, he watched her decay into obesity, prescription pills and daytime television. The young couple paid her bills and supported her.

When Ryan was growing up, his mother was seemingly oblivious about his very existence. Starting roughly when he began going to school, he was regularly bullied and his lunch money was stolen. She did not seem to notice how hungry he was when he got home, or when his clothes might be ripped or have bloodstains. Most glaringly, however, was when he haltingly told me "I was not potty trained until I was fourteen." Louise already knew about this.

Trying to contain my horror, I inquired further. Daily, year after miserable year, Ryan defecated in his pants, well into junior high school. My attempts to envision a little boy, then an adolescent trying to flee to the boys' room, washing his underwear, smelling like feces, trying to conceal the unconcealable, and being made fun of and further rejected, all of it was unfathomable. He described the nightmare of the boys' locker room, the cruel humor of the other kids, his loneliness and disgust with the mess that he felt himself to be. Most astonishing to me, was how could a mother miss this? How could she not smell or see the soiled pants and underwear, why was it not something he could tell her or his father about?

Ryan's self-disgust and revulsion against his own body and function, were congruent with his not consciously remembered rejection by his mother. He did remember how she picked up and cuddled his baby sister, who was pretty, petite and of course female. And there was a hint of sadness as he spoke of the recollection. However, seeing the whole situation as his own problem, Ryan figured out how to do his own laundry when he could, and "carried on" until the problem mysteriously "stopped." Not knowing how it stopped, however, compounded the sense of powerlessness he already felt, and his own failure of agency, which he also felt shame about. Nonetheless, Ryan cultivated a thick shell of self-reliance and did all he could for himself. He also developed an effective emotional numbing response. Later he had a series of physical ailments that called for heavy opiates which were constipating, sexually deadening and created a natural distance in the marriage.

Viewing himself as physically repulsive, smelly, inherently undesirable, and thus untouchable was an early woven-in aspect of Ryan's identity. Having this replicated in his marriage (and in a way in their previous marital therapy), was more of the same. They came to me, motivated by the Louise's chronic complaint about the drugs. As Ryan became able to wean himself from the medications, his very existence came increasingly into view. It was a long time before Ryan could speak about his sexual desire and longing, not only for sexual closeness but also for the simple experience of being physically wanted. From early on, just as the attachment literature tells us, his mother did not want to touch him. Only at the body level was Ryan able to have any remembered experience, usually activated by what felt to him like a parallel revulsion from Louise.

Cautious and painstaking somatic work, neurofeedback to help him with the fear about coming down on his meds, and deep relationship work were required. We also of course had to name the trauma of neglect. As we worked with both Louise's sexual trauma and Ryan's neglect history, he began to see the depth of trauma in his potty-training nightmare. "I think I'm a double winner," Ryan joked, meaning both trauma and neglect. Of course, we now know that is often the case.

Both peristalsis-defecation and sexuality are functions of bodily and therefore self-regulation. We now know, that the absence, insufficiency or failure of accurate mirroring, and the experience of being regulated by the primary caregiver, are inherently and fundamentally dysregulating. Ryan's symptoms reflected his profound dysregulation, and also served as powerful vehicles for communicating the largely wordless and split-off story of rejection, aloneness and the inevitable resort to a desolate substance dependence and self-reliance.

## SEXUALITY AND REGULATION

Beginning my journey toward sex therapy certification, I was surprised to learn just how wide the range is of sexual fantasy, pleasure and behavior are, and that I was much less "sexually intelligent" (hip?) than I had fancied myself to be. In turn I learned and how narrow and arbitrary the window viewed as "normal" still was and still is. Although the media bombard us with sexual imagery and titillation, we continue to be hard pressed to find and access reliable and useful sexuality information. The subject of sex still appears to be a point of shame or taboo, and ignorance, many of our clients struggle to understand. They wonder, "what is wrong with *me*?" and lack a reliable reference to measure that against, and no one safe to ask. It is "natural" so it "should" be automatic, and like in the movies, we just automatically know what our partner likes and how to "achieve" that. All the more in a self-reliant world. It is certainly anything but natural to think one would need help to ascertain what is "normal."

Attentive parents understandably worry, that now young people get their "sex education" no longer only in locker rooms or via "dirty jokes;" but on the internet and porn sites which these distressed parents often must go out of their way to block. The child of neglect will, of course, roam freely around those sites. The question of what constitutes sexual health remains largely elusive, unanswered or even un-asked. Many clients, remain mute with embarrassment or shame, and don't talk about it even with their partners, or therapists.

As we entered the 2000's the specter of so-called "Sex Addiction" burst upon the clinical and popular scene. I remember when I was in my early twenties and reading Karl Marx for the first time. His dramatic intro "A spectre is haunting Europe …" conjured images of a dark and menacing, monstrous cyclone-like cloud, sweeping up an otherwise civilized, orderly urban landscape. It was chilling. The threat of "sex addiction" came with that demonic tone. As is frequently the case in our field, there may be a "diagnosis du jour" and this unresearched and lacking in nosology or standardized definition was "dramatic," titillating and a readily frightening threat that lingered for several years.

Due to the proliferation of the internet, and readily available access for any and all variation of sexual interest, clinician Al Cooper. identified what he called the "Three A's" of "sex addiction": Accessibility, Affordability and Anonymity, and many parents, partners and even users themselves ascribed to this pathological description, and utilized the "addiction" framework, which also readily caught on. A veritable industry of "sex addiction" training and treatment mushroomed, which the official sex therapy field (the certifying body for sex therapists), fought against valiantly.

I received panicked calls from spouses or partners, or "addicts" themselves. I still see couples struggling to recover from the traumatic rupture of those times, although I rarely hear of "sex addiction" anymore, and I am not sure what became of all those specialists and treatment programs. I view this experience of compulsion or unmanageable sexual urge and behavior, as another expression of dysregulation, a lack of balance between sympathetic and parasympathetic, safety and passion. And because of my being not exclusively, but perhaps best known, as a relationship therapist, I most often encountered these clients in the context of a couple.

One such couple, Roger and Diane, came to me having been in a variety of different prior treatment settings. Not uncharacteristically, she had wanted him to be "evaluated" by a sex addiction specialist, which included a lie detector test. Roger found the assessment humiliating and insulting. He seemed to be at his breaking point with the marriage. It was true that he had had multiple brief and from her point of view, "kinky" affairs. She did not understand the kinkiness which involved costumes and scenes, rough behavior and dirty talk.

He did not want to do any of those things with her, not that she would have agreed to it. In fact, he did not want to have sex with her at all.

Diane was extraordinarily attractive. Small, exquisitely fit and trim, impeccably dressed and made up, even to come to therapy, and with the grace and poise of a prima ballerina. She was also almost shockingly angry, and her rage was searing and terrifying, as well as extremely distasteful and offensive to Roger. It made him want to withdraw dramatically, to cut and run. That was when the infidelities would occur, which just elicited another wave of rage and censure, another bout of escape, and an escalating cycle. But now she had a diagnosis and treatment plan for him.

Roger's mother left him when he was an infant. He was raised by an angry alcoholic father, but largely raised himself. His younger years were lonely and riddled with his father's long alcoholic absences. He early learned to fend for himself. In high school, he discovered long-distance running, and found in it an escape from his father's bellowing rage, a calming effect on his body, and a freedom to let his thoughts roam. And he found he was good at it, and winning and being a desired team-mate was a welcome relationship experience. Being a valued member on a team with other boys, in a primarily individual sport, was about the level of intimacy and contact that was comfortable for him, although he did not think about it that way. He just knew he liked the team, he loved running, he liked winning and being wanted for being good. And he felt empowered by having the means in his own body of escape from his father.

Roger dated little in high school. He masturbated a lot, but he was shy and awkward. When he met Diane in college, he was dazzled. She was so beautiful. And although she was immensely critical and prone to anger, that all felt so familiar to him, that he scarcely noticed it. His whole childhood had trained and desensitized him to that. Having her attention even for a minute, amazed and swept him away. Diane was also extremely busy with her own, "very important" career which meant she had precious little time or attention for him. They soon got married, got a dog and started a life together.

Roger got very close to their dog. With Diane there was always significant distance. They had sex occasionally, but he never seemed to be able to get it right for her, and she was quick to anger about that. Her angry criticism was sharp and stinging. Diane told him only once shortly after they got married, that she had experienced sexual trauma in her childhood. She never told him what happened, who, how often, how old she had been, nothing. She had never told anyone. That was one of the rare moments between them, where he got a tiny window into her vulnerability, and heart.

When I met Roger and Diane, he was an accomplished ultra-distance runner (yes another one!) He regularly completed 100-mile runs. It also seemed as if he was chronically in flight from Diane's anger and criticism, as well as her preoccupation with her career; her busy-ness, and chronic rejection of him. Roger calmed himself, regulated his nervous system with running, and later with serial affairs and sex workers. The gulf between them widened. Her criticism morphed into vicious, if understandable, suspicion. When he was out, Diane regularly examined his computer for porn sites and found plenty, and credit card bills that might expose his visits to hotels, strip clubs and escorts, which meant he was often greeted with rage and critical dramatic accusations when he came home. Between the infidelities that she was skilled at uncovering, the "hooker charges" she found on his credit card, and the prolific porn, she viewed Roger as an "addict." Roger was in fact driven and it would not have been easy for him to stop, but my view is there was another way of looking at this. Diane was also perennially and vociferously mad that he did not want to have sex with her. He viewed her rather as a praying mantis, known for eating the partner alive, after they have sex.

## OUT OF CONTROL SEXUAL BEHAVIOR

In general, lurking below the surface in clients like Roger, I often uncovered a neglect history, and a person more fluent in relationships that are distant, disconnected, lacking in emotion, intimacy, commitment and transparency. And an inability to manage the interplay between arousal and calm. Perhaps this compulsive sexuality was another way to illustrate or communicate the unconscious story of intense and unrelenting wanting, and experiencing a fleeting facsimile of being momentarily wanted. Of course, this is a gross and hypothetical oversimplification of a complex constellation of individual and interpersonal dynamics. But it was a way of conceptualizing these difficulties, especially when the client themselves, were suffering from it. Accessing those buried feelings of longing, loneliness and hopelessness became a treatment objective for me. As well as beginning to develop the first tolerance and ultimately even pleasure of connecting and being close with the partner. With Roger and Diane, it was difficult to get to enough regulation and quiet in the room to go near this vital intervention.

Braun-Harvey and Vigorito wrote eloquently about men and women like Roger and also developed a coherent, practical analysis and treatment model consisting of individual and group therapy, and couple's therapy when appropriate. They coined the term "out of control sexual behavior," (OCSB) which some clients find comforting and accurately descriptive, and others in my experience, find offensive. I found the model to be a great help to me in how I think about this particular disordered sexual expression. Continuing to find a correlation between neglect and OCSB I worked with couples to attempt to quiet the storm or bridge the gulf which they invariably seemed had burst open between them; help them to replicate the missing experience of being seen and mirrored, and teach concrete intimacy skills, verbal, nonverbal, tactile and erotic. It was certainly not quick or easy for anyone.

For Roger and Diane, it was too late, by the time they got to me. Sometimes sadly our work cannot be completed because the clients have lost too much time, and been re-injured too much to stay the course. We must have the humility to examine where we in fact did err. And learn what we can.

## THE "SAFE" DISTANCE

The theme, as we can see, is maintaining the familiar and therefore manageable distance, so as to gratify the undeniable need, and keep the fear of loss, abandonment or rejection, at bay. All of these "solutions" are in the service of that, often primitive, often quite ingenious attempts to balance two competing and powerful forces. For many a child of neglect, whose general nervous system baseline as we have seen, is "under-aroused," introducing excitement via their sexual behavior, may be a way of enlivening or awakening a flat or drowsy existence. It might include thrill seeking or even risky or dangerous behavior. Luke would frequent the park known as a hotbed for anonymous sex, during the era of the HIV/AIDS epidemic, knowing he was playing Russian Roulette. Was he enacting the extreme to which he had felt worthless and dispensable as a child? Was it a way to be intimate quickly and briefly and then escape? Was it a way to feel alive, or connect with a lost part of himself? We had to explore them all, and once we did, the behavior which was rich with meanings, was not needed anymore. Luke was amazed, (with the help of neurofeedback I must add) it "just stopped."

For Elizabeth, becoming a sex worker became a solution. She could feel desired and desirable, she could be in control, she could set all the terms herself, and not have to concern herself with emotion or mutuality. The money made her feel valued. Time and place were in her control and circumscribed. The secrecy required to be safe from moral and legal interruption was the only consideration that made sex work ultimately unsustainable beyond a certain point. But by then, she had processed enough about her neglect that she wanted to move on.

## THE "PANDEMIC" OF 2017

In 2017 our world was awakened by the "Me Too" movement, an outpouring of loud and outspoken testimonial from legions of women, breaking silence about their histories of sexual assault, harassment, exploitation and abuse of every ilk, as children or adults. As a therapist of the traumatized and a champion of the sexually violated, and of women over many decades, having these issues intrude into public awareness and rattle inertia and denial, was a tremendous and long-awaited relief. I hope the gains we made have not faded or been lost, due to their eclipse by other and similarly crucial public preoccupations, certainly in 2020.

I was infinitely gratified and hopeful, about issues of gender power imbalance and sexual social justice finally getting their due. However, as a tireless advocate for sexual health as well, something bothered me. In addition to a major social, political and moral heresy, we were staring in the face of a major public health crisis, except no one was talking about that. I kept asking myself, "what is *wrong* with these men?" Besides being opportunists, power mongers or "chauvinist pigs," as we used to say in my day, operating freely in an unjust and under-monitored power structure, these men were massively dysregulated.

The men we were hearing about, had it all, and had everything to lose by acting wantonly and stupidly. Men like Bill Clinton or Bill Cosby, were already powerful and successful. Why would they risk all that, to have sex with unconscious women, or serial seemingly meaningless flings? Granted, the problem was not limited to the rich and famous. But if, as we all were now beginning to see and hear, the scale of abuse and exploitation is this massive, in addition to the finally acknowledged corruption of power, something is amiss in the development and education of boys. In addition to having a profoundly corrupt gender power dynamic and imbalance in our culture, we have a major public health issue regarding sexual health.

As the stories came pouring forth, I listened. Sometimes the perpetrators were famous men, known to me. Often not. What had so wildly highjacked their nervous systems, that this kind of wanton recklessness and disregard, with the grave potential to wreak serious damage not only against their hapless victims but also to themselves? I did not know the histories of any of the men I was reading about, except I that I remembered years ago, having read one article about Bill Clinton's childhood. My intent was not to excuse the behavior, or pity these men, but rather to take the problem perhaps further upstream. I had also heard a smattering of pain and shame ridden disclosures from my neglect clients, who in a maximally dysregulated time in their lives, or while in the haze of substance abuse, had done similarly unforgivable things. This is not to suggest that our neglect clients are necessarily perpetrators of any kind, or pathological. But rather, that attachment trauma and its attendant dysregulations, in addition to touch deprivation, are a potent elixir with many possible results. Most often it is a powerful longing and physical and emotional loneliness that accompany unconscious fear and grief. But there are plenty of other expressions.

Wrestling with these ideas, I wrote an article about them that I posted on my website. Ironically, I gave it as a title, a word that in 2017, was not yet the household word it has since become. Ironically, I called my article, "Pandemic." And I do believe, even if the centrality in the news is not the same as it was, the problem has not gone away, but continues urgent, even amidst other critically urgent social outcry. As long as the dysregulations continue, the intergenerational transmission of trauma persists, and so also do all of its insidious reverberations.

This other Pandemic, underscores and emphasizes my passion about healing the dysregulations so they go no further; and of providing quality, frank and evidence-based sex education for boys and girls (and parents for that matter); an understanding of sexual health; what constitutes "normal" sexuality, and what sorts of impulses and even sensations, might require containment or even treatment. Making this sort of educational information available and accessible is a neglected public health matter, as is healing the dysregulations of trauma, developmental trauma, and within that neglect.

I remember from when I was two, waking up terrified from dreams of "army men" running loudly through the house, overturning tables and waste baskets, stuffing bags with whatever was around, waving guns. It was my mother's nightmare, my mother's unhealed and unprocessed trauma. The nature of trauma is to re-enact it in some explicit or implicit way, until it is processed, healed and turns to something else.


## SEXUAL HEALTH

Attitudes, norms, information, values and sex education, have always been colored and shaped by prevailing political trends and attitudes. In 2001, the enlightened then-Surgeon General, Dr. David Satcher issued a "Call to Action to Promote Sexual Health and Responsible Sexual Behavior." Partly in response or reaction to the crises of HIV and AIDS, and teen pregnancy, it was a political time of greater receptivity. It was also a far cry from the culture of "pussy grabbing," and expensive escorts with gag orders, that have been the culture of recent times. Children of neglect, always at a loss for guidance and direction, in this world of sexuality, are again thrown on their own resources to make sense of an essential, complex, elusive and unavoidable aspect of life.

Braun-Harvey and Vigorito identified the Six Principles of Sexual Health, which are simple, precise and easy to teach. They embody dignity and respect, and place value on relationship; while also inviting a wide berth of diversity, inclusivity and acceptance: a breath of fresh air, in these deceit-ridden times. I like to teach the six principles to couples and clients, especially children of neglect, to begin to dismantle the shame and self-rejection of feeling sexually pathological or dysfunctional, and having internalized their early experience of body rejection that way. And also, to address their confusion about what is "OK" to do or want to do; or simply the perennial and often dreaded question of, *what to do*. Granted much more is required to alter such deep, and often preverbal experience, but I find the principles useful, and perhaps empowering, nonetheless.

The Six Principles of Sexual Health as spelled out so elegantly by Braun Harvey and Vigorito are the following:

- Consent.
- Non-exploitation.
- Honesty.
- Shared values.
- Protection from STI, HIV and unwanted pregnancy.
- Mutual pleasure.

Each of the principles may require a rich amount of discussion about what they mean; and to "practice" those discussions with the therapist can be enlightening, as well as continue to "exercise the muscle" of talking explicitly about sexual matters. Partners will have much to agree on; what constitutes consent, exploitation, shared values and even pleasure, let alone mutual pleasure? Beyond these non-negotiables, personal taste and fantasy is unlimited. Individuals and couples can freely decide together, what to *do*, sexually.

Within these principles, specific sexual activities are secondary. And having clear parameters help with fears and beliefs, that "there is something wrong with you," and/or "There is something wrong with me."

## SUMMING UP AND WHAT TO DO

- We have examined the mere tip of a veritable personal and cultural iceberg, and of course a bare peek (no pun intended!) at the innumerable variations of dysregulated or alienated sexuality we may encounter. Because sexuality inhabits the interface between attachment, regulation and the emotional and somatic experience of the body, all epicenters of utmost significance for our neglect clients, it is essential that we address it. Every one of us has a sex life, whether completely internal and wished for, or actually lived, in real time. We must take this as given. Some clients may have made their peace with whatever their expression is or has been, including asexuality. Others may live with grief and even anger, about lost time and missed experience, the loneliness of skin hunger or touch deprivation, or body hatred. They may feel robbed or cheated. They may suffer from shame about their "ignorance," about something so primitive and innate; about having more rejections, about betrayals of others, about their bodies, about disrespect they may have tolerated or accepted, about mistreatment of themselves. I view the work with sexuality through the triumvirate lens of attachment, regulation and psychoeducation.

- Sexuality spoken here: let the client know that you are open, interested and able to invite this taboo subject into the open. Get fluent and even practice saying the words aloud comfortably: penis, vagina, masturbate, clitoris, etc. You want to model an ease about including these topics in our work, without the shame that is shrouded behind euphemism or metaphor. And use their language: if they say "get it on" or "horny" use their word, unless of course they are self-deprecating or demeaning of anyone.

- Provide accurate education: Teach the Six Principles of Sexual Health. Invite questions and if you don't know the answers, be transparent about that and have the humility to find out for them This also helps direct their attention away from ever consulting the internet, which as we know is often a questionable, values/marketing laden "consultant." This means assembling resources and resource people with whom you can consult with confidence.

- Place sexuality squarely in a regulation framework, which by the time we become able to talk about sex, they have understanding about. This is both normalizing and perhaps engenders hope, as they may see an access route for working on sexuality that they have not seen before.

- Be aware of your "ick factors," the sexual acts that evoke a horror, outrage, disgust or incredulity in yourself. The American Association of Sex Educators, Counselors and Therapists (AASECT) which is the sex therapist certification body, and a foremost source of reliable education and training, offers a Sexual Attitude Reassessment (SAR), the first required step toward Sex Therapist certification. It is an intense several-day workshop. (My first one was seven 12-hour days long, in a picturesque mountain setting, which became affectionately referred to as "Sex Camp.") Experience of being exposed to a wide variety of possible sexual expressions that we may or may not have even imagined, discussing and processing our reactions to them, even speaking with others about our own sexual fantasy and practice. Its intention is to bring to awareness and neutralize our "ick factors" so we won't meet the client with revulsion. It may be a valuable (even fun) Continuing Education endeavor!

- Check your own judgments and attitudes about pornography and the client engaging with sex workers. Given attachment difficulties, or the default to self-reliance or a sexual configuration that is unrelated or independent of a live and reciprocal other, this is not unusual.

- Sexuality being rich with meanings (and for some morals, that may surprise you), be curious and inquiring about those also. These conversations can be both powerful and connecting, as well as enlightening.

- As ever address the attachment component, whether it be about a relationship they are recounting, or family of origin attachment experiences. And continue to provide that missing experience of presence, consistency, seeing and hearing them and who they are.

- Model comfort in your own skin if possible, and be as candid and vocal as is natural and authentic for you about acceptance of their bodies, of course being exquisitely mindful of a clear and ever-present safe boundary between you.

- Inquire about touch in the family, being breastfed, held, in an incubator, left alone, anything remembered or that they might have learned later about their early life. If they are isolated recommend massage therapy. Of course, as I write this, everything is circumscribed by COVID, so we are all painfully touch deprived. I have faith that will end some day!

- Utilize whatever somatic methodologies you practice, or make appropriate referrals. Educate yourself about which of the available websites offer resources and activities for clients that are consonant with your approach. There are many out there that are good and also free of charge.

- Be mindful to find the delicate balance: not villainizing the parent (or partner); contextualizing behavior (when appropriate) as making sense in light of the attachment narrative; and introducing hope and optimism.

- If there is a partner, and you are working with the individual, recommend couple's therapy with a good sex positive and trauma-informed couple's therapist. This means having a reserve of known, competent and trustworthy referrals whose approach is compatible with your own.
- Continue the work of regulation, whatever modality that means for you.
- Be clearly and explicitly sex positive and relaxed; interested and curious (but not "*too*" much); non-judgmental and open-minded; educated and broadly informed.
- This is not a cookbook, and we will find more variations than we ever imagined. Like cheese making, although all the recipes begin with the same one ingredient, gross and subtle differences, (some intended and some idiosyncratic or mistaken) of cooking time, temperature, micro amounts of bacteria and age, give us the over three thousand varieties of cheese that the world enjoys. So, we must be flexible and willing to learn all the time.
- Sexuality resides at the interfaces between body, nervous system/brain and relationship; and also regulation, attachment and somatic experience of the self. In effect it hits at the core of all the major areas of vulnerability to the child of neglect. So it merits our attention, and often commands it. And yes, much of the time we will gently, non-coercively and with painstaking consent, have to "coax it out" of the client. This means practicing the Six Principles in our process!
- Implicit here of course, but worth saying explicitly, we therapists must attend to our own sexual issues! Yes, we do have them too!

## BIBLIOGRAPHY

Carroll, Joe. "Clinton's Wife Says He Was 'Scarred by Abuse' as a Child." *Irish Times*, August 2, 1999. https://www.irishtimes.com/news/clinton-s-wife-says-he-was-scarred-by-abuse-as-child-1.212700.

Cassidy, Jude, and Phillip R. Shaver, eds. *Handbook of Attachment: Theory, Research, and Clinical Application.* 3rd ed. New York: The Guilford Press, 2016.

Cohn, Ruth. *Coming Home to Passion: Restoring Loving Sexuality in Couples with Histories of Childhood Trauma and Neglect. Sex, Love, and Psychology.* Santa Barbara, California: Praeger, 2011.

Cohn, Ruth. "Toward a Trauma-Informed Approach to Adult Sexuality: A Largely Barren Field Awaits Its Plow." *Current Sexual Health Reports* 8, no. 2 (April 2016): 77–85. https://doi.org/10.1007/s11930-016-0071-4.

Cooper, Al, ed. "Cybersex: The Dark Side of the Force." *Special issue, Sexual Addiction and Compulsivity: The Journal of Treatment and Prevention* 7, no. 1–2: 285. (August 2000).

Decker, Julie Sondra. *The Invisible Orientation: An Introduction to Asexuality.* New York: Skyhorse, 2015.

Douglas, Braun-Harvey, and Michael A. Vigorito. *Treating out of Control Sexual Behavior: Rethinking Sex Addiction.* New York: Springer, 2016.

Hendrix, Harville. *Getting the Love You Want: A Guide for Couples.* 20th anniversary ed. New York: Henry Holt, 2008.

Luker, Kristin. *When Sex Goes to School: Warring Views on Sex—and Sex Education—since the Sixties.* New York: W. W. Norton, 2006.

Maltz, Wendy. *The Sexual Healing Journey: A Guide for Survivors of Sexual Abuse.* 3rd ed. New York: HarperCollins, 2012.

McNaught, Brian. *Sex Camp.* Bloomington, Indiana: AuthorHouse, 2005.

O'Loughlin, Julia I., Alessandra H. Rellini, and Lori A. Brotto. "How Does Childhood Trauma Impact Women's Sexual Desire? Role of Depression, Stress, and Cortisol." *Journal of Sex Research* 57, no. 7 (September 2020): 836–847. https://doi.org/10.1080/00224499.2019.1693490.

Satcher, David. "The Surgeon General's Call to Action to Promote Sexual Health and Responsible Sexual Behavior." *American Journal of Health Education* 32, no. 6 (December 2001): 356–368. https://doi.org/10.1080/19325037.2001.10603498.

# Regulation of Giving: From Resentment to Reciprocity

Infancy is the one and probably only time in our lives, when reciprocity is not expected or even possible. It is similarly perhaps the only time when the fabled "unconditional love" is a realistic wish. Nature designed babies to be so adorable and oxytocin to be so intoxicating as to inspire the impulse to regale the child with a flow of whatever it is, they might need; and to facilitate a bond. This is nature's plan, supporting the imperative to preserve the species. We have a primal need, to be welcomed and received, even if it is not always what comes to pass, for a host of possible reasons.

When neglect begins from the start, as with many of our clients it probably does, although it is hard to know for sure, this one-time opportunity is missed, or is deficient at best. Regardless of when it begins, however, the primary experience of neglect is to be *ungratified*. The fundamental need is unmet. Besides being dysregulating, this is painful and confusing, and engenders the initial question: the unanswerable *why*? Which, along with its shapeshifting answers, is also likely to be unconscious.

The next question for the child is perhaps more a challenge than a question: *how* can I secure some sort of glue between us? If I can't inherently elicit or "merit" connection, is there a way to earn it, buy it, barter for it? Or somehow compensate for whatever the "answer" is to the unanswerable why? Searching for such a strategy, as the default to self-reliance coagulates, becomes a way to survive. In the course of it, dynamics of giving and receiving in general, and most markedly receiving, become complex and fraught.

This chapter will examine some of the labyrinthine dynamics surrounding giving and receiving. Both sides of the equation contain numerous, often conflicting emotions, beliefs, personal "rules," practices and assumptions about self and other, providing another window into the client's interpersonal world. We will also consider, what are the gains versus costs of their particular strategy? What their fears and hopes might be, about changing something about it? And how the therapeutic relationship as ever, provides a stage both where dynamics are revealed, and possibly for experimenting with something different.

## "THE PERFECT WAITER": SHAME AND PURPOSE

The strategies that children of neglect create may be elaborate and brilliant. They may also be so adaptive as to translate into later assets in other areas of their lives. This again, is double edged. The pain underneath will be out of view, which is in some ways preferable. But in others it masks the reality of the child's lonely existence, and in effect contributes to the invisibility of their authenticity. This double-edged-ness, may make this tangle all the more complicated to examine. The client's question may well then be, "well what is wrong with that?" meaning, "This strategy works for me, well sort of …" And "sort of" might seem better than nothing, which may also make change somewhat risky. This as any other behavior change, or relinquishing of a known and long utilized strategy may seem to threaten them with more loss, or leave them feeling defenseless and back at sea.

Lois created a paradigm she rather affectionately called the "Perfect Waiter." The perfect waiter anticipates what the customer wants, even before that customer is aware of wanting it, and fulfills the need or wish so quickly and seamlessly as to not even to be seen doing it. The napkin is replaced folded, the bread basket refilled, the wine poured, as if by elves in the night. Lois prided herself in it, and it served her well. It later served her well again in real restaurants, when she was working her way through college and graduate school.

Lois's mother's anxiety was such that anticipating and fulfilling her needs, before she herself experienced them gnawing at her, "was a way both to keep myself safe, and to exist." Safe in that when Lois's mother was anxious, she was angry, critical, sometimes violent or "she simply left." By managing her mother's states, Lois had a modicum of control over her environment; and it afforded her some measure of "shalom bayit," peace in the house. In Lois's somewhat traditional Jewish family, shalom bayit was a cherished family value, that sadly, rarely existed as more than just that, a valued perhaps mysterious aspiration. Still, Lois's belief that she might be contributing to or enhancing a semblance of family peace, was another point of pride, as well as that smidgeon of safety.

"Even if it was not noticed, being the perfect waiter seemed to give me a purpose. I could quietly help. Even if she was not aware of it, my mom had a better day. I helped her have a better day. I had silently made the house a little cleaner, made her bed, washed the breakfast dishes. It quieted the storm a bit. I guess I did that too," and Lois herself also had a better day. "Great service" also seemed to provide some justification for being, or a morsel of self-worth. "At least I had *that* to offer in a way I guess it made me a pretty good deal." Except for the daily cost or blight of her existence. In effect Lois believed she had been earning her keep, making the "deal" worth it for her mom. It is important to note, even in the somewhat proud, cute, even idyllic little waiter story, told with a smile, that the down side lurks not far under the blithe surface. It sounded rather like indentured servitude, and she could not afford to let up.

Lois's predominant and default, chronic feelings were "invisible and worthless," Shame was ambient air to her, the only sense of self she had ever known. She was less aware of the fear. When she was old enough to go to school, these feelings all went with her. There she was a bright, solitary and with all of that going on inside, sad little girl.

The perfect waiter became a sense of self to Lois. Without even realizing it, in whatever relationships she managed to have, Lois replicated some form of this pattern. Always the themes of neglect reappeared: worthlessness, not feeling entitled to exist; needing to earn the bit of ground she occupied on the planet or in the other's day; compensating for her unsavory existence; not knowing what else to do to exist in the eyes of the other. She desperately feared she would vanish if she stopped "serving" although when she was not doing it, if she dared to stop for a minute, she hid, not knowing who to be.

On some level Lois also harbored a secret wish, that these superior efforts to be thoughtful would secure her some measure of specialness, an ironic contrast to the assumption of invisibility. To be noticed, was somehow not enough. It was more than just "breaking even," she wanted to be the *most* special, to be chosen over the rest. It was her unique version of all or nothing. Either she was nonexistent, or "perfect." Admittedly it was exhausting, and not really effective.

Invariably, eventually, the "perfect waiter" was taken for granted, or being unseen "got old." The other had all the power, and that would become tiring. Gradually, and in spite of herself, she would start noticing subtle blasts of bitterness, and come to resent and take issue with the imbalance of give and take. If she raised it to the unwitting other, they might be surprised and feel as if she was suddenly presenting a bill for something they never asked for. Granted they had received and even possibly enjoyed what she provided. But they would feel trapped or blindsided. That was when her relationships usually self-destructed. And the littered path of failed relationships that trailed behind her, only added to her well of shame.

Of course, Lois brought these assumptions and practices into the relationship with me. She was scrupulously mindful of our ending time making sure to be out the door before I might need to end the session. She paid me ahead, so fearful of overstaying her welcome, or simply not being worth the trouble. She thanked me for everything. "Thank you for your hospitality!" she would say. I knew I needed to watch and listen, and anticipate, being on a careful lookout for opportunities to work with her on how her resentment might play out between us. Or if she was feeling with me already, that her specialness didn't count, or didn't "work." or if there was already a bit of this indenturedness happening. Being cautious, I hoped would contribute to Lois's experience of feeling seen and heard, and perhaps help prevent my becoming part of the litter pile. It may I considered, also be frightening.

Lois told me a story of a previous therapist she had had. She had given the therapist a gift of a beautiful, artfully tiled, expensive hand mirror. She thought a mirror was a clever gift for a therapist, and this therapist was an "artistic type" who Lois imagined would respond to the aesthetic aspect, the beauty of it, and also see that Lois had spent a lot of money on her. She was excited and really believed this gift would "mean something." When Lois presented the artistically wrapped gift, the therapist unwrapped it graciously, but her response was muted, an "uneventful, quiet thank you." Lois was crushed. When she awkwardly, perhaps timidly came to her session the following week, she was confused about how to feel. Hurt, mad? She just did not understand. Did the therapist just not "like" the gift?

At this point in the telling, Lois, flustered, could not even remember what she had said to the therapist, it was some sort of inquiry about how the therapist liked the gift. She did, however, remember the therapist's response: "I like it fine," she said. "I just don't want you to think you have to do things like that for me." Obviously, this therapist was trying in her way, to work with Lois's impulse to give or over-give, in her attempt to earn or buy love. Lois did not remember how she had felt, "mostly shame, I think. I quit that therapist that day. Never went back." In this story was perhaps a warning to me, or a plea. If stripped of the defense too soon, she would be rudderless, and terrified.

Fortunately, Lois stayed the course, It was a delicate business to broach the giving patterns with her, Her brittle construction of this painstaking insurance of acceptability in the eye of another, particularly someone important in her attachment system, was her lifeline. Without it, she was lost in a stormy sea. It was safer to remain invisible, than to lose the only person she knew how to be. And putting language to her self-hatred would be humiliating at best.

The therapist must remain astute, both about the giving, and the delicacy of how we address it. And too, we must stay mindful about the big and little perks we get from her their perhaps excessive attentiveness. They may in fact be tantalizingly convenient, labor-saving or simply seamlessly easy to miss. It is a bit of a break when the client manages her own time, or is thoughtful or considerate of us. We must not like it "too much." We must at the very least remain mindful of it, being aware of when the client goes above and beyond, and naming it, acknowledging and if appropriate, appreciating it. Just naming it may connote that their act was "more" than the norm. And above all, we are keeping them visible, and not in danger of vanishing, at least in our eyes. It is a powerful process.

Of course, there are also times when I choose to cautiously prevent or block the over-giving behavior. The perfect waiter also tracks and remembers the customer's name, tastes and preferences, her grandchildren's names and the details of their last conversation; to be able to thoughtfully follow up. Lois would practice this kind of thoughtfulness with everyone, inquiring caringly about this and about that, until all the time was taken up and there was no time for her to talk about herself. Then she would lament that she was invisible and "no one asked" her about herself. She was puzzled about this. "Why do grocery store checkers always seem to tell me their life stories while I am checking out in the grocery line? What is it about me? It is not like they *ever* ask me about how I am!" Here was a safe and splendid invitation to explore.

> "Most people love talking about themselves," I told her. "Given the opportunity they will, and they may go on and on. And all the more because you are an extraordinary listener." Cautiously aware of her ready default to self-blame, or readiness to hear me as if I am saying it is her "fault," I added, "I won't let you disappear yourself with me." I learned to be very spare in my answers to her questions about myself, not shutting her out, but protecting her, from her own tendency. We all have our own clinical stance and personal style about self-disclosure with our clients. With children of neglect, I am particularly inten- tional about where I draw my line. My typical tendency is to be fairly and cautiously loose, especially as I get older and feel more "liberty" for whatever reason. And now during COVID that I am working from home, they can see a bit of where I live on the screen. With some children of neglect, this is very meaningful. With others, like Lois, I cut it very short, "enough about me! Tell me about you!"

When Lois and I did start speaking of our relationship, at first it was unimaginable to her that what we were in was a relationship; and what is more that she was quite acceptable and even worthy of care, without extraordinary effort, without doing more than everyone else, or being "perfect, whatever that is." She simply could not believe it. Eventually, we were able to contact first the complaint, then the anger, and eventually the grief about how impoverished her childhood had been, and how tiring the barter system, and the waitering had been. It took very much longer to truly believe it was not her "fault."

I might add, that Lois was extremely intelligent and well defended, meaning her prefrontal cortex, her rational brain was where she operated from most, which is a blessing and a curse. She was well read and could regularly "figure out" what was going on psychologi- cally, which did not change much. She was less able to contact emo- tion. But one way that Lois made herself "special" which actually served her, was that she was always ready and willing to be a "guinea pig" with new modalities I had learned. Even when I was the only one in town doing this "beeping cure," neurofeedback, which no one out here had ever heard of, she was delighted to be one of my first to try it out. The neurofeedback, facilitated access to much more feeling, and greatly accelerated our work. She loved it.

Cautiously after beginning to talk about her giving, about our relationship and adding neurofeedback, Lois slowly became able to experiment in other relationships, with being more measured or regulated in her giving. She realized she did not want to barter for crumbs or view herself as so unworthy anymore. She could even begin to see in a few select friendships, that when she relaxed a bit around all that doing, she did not evaporate, and that those were the relationships that were worth it *to her*.

I do alert people, that when they do deep work on themselves, "people get left behind." Lois agreed. About all those "takers," she might just be losing interest. As significant as the discovery of losing interest, was her ability to feel and register her own preference. "Wow!" she said. "I can even feel what I want! Who *is* this person?"


## DEALS, BEHOLDEN-NESS AND GIVING THE "WRONG THING"

In a one-person world, it may not occur to an individual to speak about what is in their head. Coming from a world where there was nobody there, there was no one to tell. If now there might be, it is not a natural impulse, and besides "who cares? I mean, who wants to know anyway?" So whatever personal economy, ways of being and specifically assumptions about relationship, including norms about giving, and receiving might be exquisitely coherent and clear to themselves, but never articulated to the other involved, completely unsaid.

My client Aaron, knew he was very sensitive about broken agreements. That it really "burned" him when someone defaulted on their end of a bargain. He did not know why, but Aaron was not particularly interested in things like that. He was less aware, however, of the numerous agreements that he carried unarticulated in his private universe, that the other party did not know they were in. That did capture his interest.

Aaron was a successful earner and a smart investor. He was generous to a fault, and prided himself in providing well for his children, now adults, and every partner he had ever had including both of his wives. It was his second wife with whom he came to therapy with me. What we all came to understand, including Aaron himself, was the unspoken barter system he operated under. By providing essentially everything material the other could want or need, he was entitled to

whatever he wanted, which with his wife, was primarily sexual. And it
also bought him a free ticket: it meant he could be unconcerned,
even oblivious to her sexual tastes and preferences, desires, libido
and timing. Needless to say, although happy to receive the bounty of
his generosity, Aaron's wife was more than displeased with the sexual
arrangement (that she did not know she had signed up for). The
result was endless conflict and fighting about sex, each of them
staunchly self-righteous, and believing the problem was sex. Aaron's
wife just simply could not comprehend why her husband had no
interest in her orgasm, or any of the kinds of tender erotic touch that
she had told him hundreds of times, that she longed for. In other
ways, she thought he loved her. Why not that way? Was he just not
attracted to her? And while he thought of himself as a really sexual
guy, what kind of really sexual guy, especially someone who seemed
so sensitive in other ways, would be such a one-sided lover? She was
incensed by what she experienced as aggression, coercion and a failure of consent. It made her not want to have sex with him at all. That
enraged him, and frankly this was hardly a lot to ask, in light of "all
that he did for her." Both felt a profound sense of injustice.

But Aaron had essentially the same unspoken deal with his kids,
simply with a different currency. As long as he endlessly gratified
them, mostly with money, he insured a prominent place for himself
in their lives. He had another deal with his employer, others with his
friends. It is just that no one knew they were in them. Underneath it
all, was Aaron's conviction that the only way to get love was to buy
it, or to create indebtedness where it is then the love is somehow
"owed." His childhood feelings of rejection, of being unwanted and
abandoned, were deeply buried. But he did not care to talk about
his past. His mother was in his words, angry and narcissistic; his
father "working or sleeping, and then he died. That's it." It was all
distasteful to recall. He preferred to reside in the present, and preferably just get everyone to abide by his agreements, which to him
were most reasonable.

It did pique his interest to realize both that he had an elaborate
trade agreement in his private world, and that his deals had not
been negotiated, or agreed on outside his head. He was also actually
curious himself, to unpack what the deals actually were. He was
vaguely aware of what felt "fair" to him, but not really.

Aaron discovered that part of his admittedly unconscious failure
to explicitly negotiate these deals or at least voice them aloud, was

the assumption, that probably no one would choose to participate. He had felt profoundly rejected by his absent mother, and rejection was his dreaded and feared expectation. Unwittingly he had discovered that he could effectively lure the other with goods and services, into being with him. It was a revelation to that his extreme reaction to what he experienced as broken agreements, was two-fold: he both felt rejected by the failure of the other to acknowledge, or in is system, "appreciate" what he had dutifully provided; and even worse perhaps, his system or his strategy was failing, which might leave him alone in the world. That would be devastating, and brought him dangerously close to the unprocessed feelings about his father's death, which he really did not want to visit just now.

Aaron's wife Maureen was delighted and enlightened by Aaron's engaging with the therapy and truly digging in to this looping struggle that they continually found themselves in. She loved Aaron and was immensely grateful for all he did and had done for her. She hated how others seemed to take him for granted. She did not want to seem to him to be one of them. Maureen wanted Aaron to feel appreciated and wanted. She had noticed that when there was plenty of sex, there was always enough money for whatever she wanted. And when there wasn't much sex happening, or they were in the agonizing, cycling, fight about it, suddenly money was tight.

Maureen was very much the therapy person. She had been hoping for Aaron to become more enthusiastic about our sessions, which she had only vaguely understood as another of those countless things "he did for her." It made her happy that he had found a way that our work could actually be of use "to him." Maureen also loved Aaron, revealing more of himself, which made her feel closer to him, and which stoked her sexual flame. That made him happy, and a positive loop was in play. She found the sexual agreement, not exactly what she would have chosen, made enough sense to her, that she could participate more open heartedly, which seemed to make Aaron, more sensitive to her wishes.

This is a wonderful sounding story, and yet often it takes more than one repetition to change a longstanding pattern, even a "present time" expression of it. But Aaron's growing self-awareness; the way that therapy could actually make a difference that would change his life for the better; but most of all, having someone in a caretaker role take the time to see and understand him, brought a welcome *calm* to is ordinarily highly anxious nervous system. This indicated to us all, that Aaron was processing deeply. And with or without his awareness, such emotional/somatic experience of relief, would provide impetus for him to return to therapy.

One more thing that Aaron learned that was of use to him: In addition to his unspoken trade agreements, he immensely believed his assumptions about Maureen. When he bought her expensive, sexy shoes, which he himself loved, and seeing her in them was a turn-on for him, he expected her to be thrilled. Although it was true that Maureen loved shoes, and expensive shoes were great, she already felt like a sex object to Aaron, so she invariably found a way to decline his gift of shoes, which felt rejecting to him. He learned that the deal would fail indeed if the currency was "wrong." Another good reason for speaking out loud, rather than single-handedly, or in his self-reliant habit, figuring it all out himself. One of the great tasks of neglect recovery is to "get a voice," even include the other. Aaron was beginning to learn about how that would benefit him.

## GIVING FOR A LIVING: THE CHILD OF NEGLECT AS PROFESSIONAL CAREGIVER

There are also many cases where the client has chosen a profession that both attracts and takes advantage of their reflexive and well-honed to impulse to give. There is a reason why grocery clerks and Uber drivers spill their life stories and intimate secrets to Lois. She is exceptionally attentive, and it is so natural for her to give herself generously as a receptacle, that she does not even notice that she invites it. As much as it wears her out sometimes, there is something flattering or gratifying about being the person whom everyone seems to pick out to confide in. And certainly, she was that one of her siblings. So even though she came to feel trapped, and then enraged by it, it proffered some frazzled thread of connection and specialness, until it didn't.

I not infrequently encounter neglect survivors who are in caregiving occupations, most notably nurses, doctors, not infrequently therapists. Sometimes, especially when they are doctors, they have chosen a highly regarded profession that might make the neglectful parent proud. That impetus largely fails. The devoted professional caregiver, like the perfect waiter may be rewarded for (while expected to be) the tireless martyr-like gratify-er of the other, which may make it both challenging to tease apart, and also change. They may just not want to "give that up," understandably. Nor do we want them to think they are supposed to, in order to heal. However, the healing process does bring surprises.

Jackie, whom we are now getting to know, had made a long and brilliant career in a caregiving profession. Not only was she highly skilled but also she was well loved and appreciated at work, for the first and only time ever. Understandably, work became her world. It was her version of a "social life," as it involved interaction with other people all day long. It kept her busy, and free of the unbearable lonely expanse of unstructured time and depression which had been her lonely childhood. It kept her, at least until she got home exhausted and depleted, away from the refrigerator. She was valued, and well paid. It really was an identity and an existence. Jackie loved her work and imagined she would never retire.

As she recovered, Jackie surprised herself finding she was getting, well, sick of it; and even starting to imagine a different life. Something she had never before considered. She was intrigued by the idea of a life that cast her more in the role of "nourish-ee," the receiver of the gratification. She became curious about how she might enjoy spending her time. Before COVID she had begun traveling and realizing how big the world is. On organized tours, she discovered she did not have to have friends to travel with, to be able to go, but even more, she made new friends. People liked her, even when she was not taking care of them. It was a revelation. She felt ready to take on the challenge of two-way, mutual, give and take friendships. They seemed possible to her now. Jackie realized she would ultimately retire. There were other kinds of pleasure, self-worth and ways to be appreciated. As this sank in, she found herself less and less depressed, more and more content. She liked cooking, but did not care that much about eating anymore, and was not afraid of it.

## STRIVING FOR AGENCY IN A SEA OF HELPLESSNESS

"At sea" seems a fitting image for a helpless infant, unable to awaken a response to its need from the caregiver. When being cute, or crying fail, the infant is helpless and lacks options, other than collapse. There is nothing to be done, but wait. The void of waiting feels deathly. When action fails, no alternative action remains, it is traumatic, the overstimulation of despair remains remembered by the undeveloped emotional and somatic brain. Interpersonal need becomes a dreaded enemy, disavowed and avoided as soon as humanly possible. So, we must stay mindful, that receiving, which if gratifying might dangerously awaken the safely stowed and buried traumatic interpersonal need, and any accompanying emotion. Tied to survival, it may be accompanied by a terror or profound urgency. We cannot take this lightly.

In turn, for someone like Aaron, the reflex to reach for the restaurant bill, even the deal making, may also be a much-needed gesture of agency, of initiating intentional purposeful action in the interpersonal world. It may be the only medium he thinks he has for securing attachment of any kind, even if many of his relationships are less than satisfying. Giving that up, even examining it, will be a long-term undertaking for Aaron. He can accept sex from Maureen as it is in accord with his safe system. That he is receptive to the therapy, and having it be more than to "fix" Maureen, is a huge step for him. We must hold this in mind.

We are most able to identify that giving and over-giving as a first-line defense, are wearing thin, when the client is clearly getting sick of it. Jackie was explicitly aware that she was getting sick of caregiving, and was getting closer to being ready and able to slough it off. Lois was aware of resentment for a long time, so we monitor her readiness to actually address this. Resentment is so distasteful, that for some, once aware of it, learning to process and eliminate it, becomes attractive.

Some of our neglect clients, espouse the label "co-dependent" which I am not fond of, as it seems to hold a critical, judgmental and pathologizing view of a person who is invested, perhaps overly so, and somewhat compulsively, about caregiving and being needed. In the 12-Step lexicon, resentment is viewed as toxic. Whatever the association, resentment is an access route, for beginning to address and change the over-giving tendency. I teach clients that we are each responsible to regulate our own giving. If I over-give and then resent, it is my own doing, or as a loudly teach, "If I over-give and then resent, it is on me!" I cannot blame the recipient. It becomes an exercise in agency, which is also ultimately empowering and gratifying.

A word about client gifts: for some clients, a way to exist or be special is by giving the therapist things. I know it was for me in my earliest days, when I could not believe or fathom that I could be remembered without leaving something to represent me. It reminds me of the way my dad joked about how he had shared a bed with so many people, that when he went to the bathroom in the night, he had to leave a bookmark. I needed both to leave some evidence, and also mark for myself, that I had a space to return to. My therapist was incredibly gracious about it, and modeled a flexibility about both giving and receiving gifts from and to me. Different therapists have a range both of ethical boundary, clinical approach and personal style. I recommend thinking this through ahead, and having a stance on it, whatever yours is, you will need to process it carefully and gently, as it may occur.

Gifts can also provide a rich clinical vein to mine. Lois once gave me a gift of a little pin she had gotten from her mother. Her mother had such a bad "rap" in our therapy, that she wanted me to have something pretty from her mom. The following week when she came back, she was anxious, scared, defensive and even a rather aggressive. She urgently wanted it back. Of course, I returned it to her. Then she was ashamed. She could not believe she had done that. She felt somehow like I was stealing her mom from her, or her mom's goodness. And she also felt like a "bad person" for reclaiming her stolen property.

She subsequently remembered and told me, a horrible childhood memory. Her mother frequently had given her things and then taken them back. And how painful that was for her. She never knew what she could safely receive or enjoy, and she also never knew quite why her mother had given or taken back the item in question. It was yet another of the unanswerables, that made giving and receiving so complicated for Lois. She needed that story to find its way out, so we could work on that painful memory, which clearly made giving and receiving more complicated for her.

## SUMMING UP AND WHAT TO DO

- The unmistakable, consistent presence of the therapist is the most invaluable of "gifts," however thankless for a very long time.
- Be aware that giving and receiving are likely to be areas of vulnerability to hold in mind, especially as gift-giving occasions like birthdays and holidays approach.

- Inquire about gifts and birthdays in the childhood home. What it was like to give. What if anything they got. Anything they can remember about that. Track carefully for emotion.
- If they are partnered, how do they handle money, sharing versus separateness in their relationship. Who pays for what, and who owns what?
- What might they feel about "sharing" versus "giving?" Sometimes while giving may feel safe and empowering, and re-enforce agency and autonomy; sharing may activate a scarcity nerve, a fear of not getting "enough."
- Listen carefully for resentment. It may be difficult to hear at first. As ever, stay attentive.
- If you suspect the neglect started very young, cognitive memory will not be available, and whatever memory there is will be somatic and/or emotional. Your non-verbal modalities and skills will be helpful.
- I often find it evocative, to imagine aloud, an infant "at sea," i.e. alone and not getting a response to their most primitive needs; and after trying to bring the caregiver back, the inevitable default to despair, collapse and ultimately self-reliance. If they have a child, you might frame it in an image of their little one, "at sea." An emotional response is often stirred by such images. I might even recommend they look for the videos of Ed Tronick's Still Face experiments, which illustrate how quick and intense an infant's reaction will be to no response.
- Be prepared for the possibility that they will want/attempt to give or over-give to you.
- Stay attentive to your own giving and receiving with these clients, so as not to slip into any re-enactment with them, around fees, time, "specialness" or some other variation.
- Introduce the notion that receiving, and receiving with gratitude, are acts of humility and courage, even generosity. Both being qualities that they generally both take pride in and value.
- Be attentive for pangs of resentment in yourself, feeling overly depleted, taxed or somehow less gratified, signals of your own over-giving.

- Giving and receiving may be complex and potentially extremely productive areas for work with neglect clients. They may also be profoundly delicate and survival related, so we must proceed with caution. Relationship work often makes clients' patterns easier to see, but they will most likely show up eventually with the therapist.
- Having non-verbal modalities as part of their therapy is always a plus, especially if we suspect the neglect began very early which it often did. Autobiographical, or "semantic" memory, simply will not have been laid down yet.

## BIBLIOGRAPHY

Alcoholics Anonymous. *Alcoholics Anonymous.* 4th ed. United States: Alcoholics Anonymous World Services Inc., 2001. First published in 1939.

# Chapter 8

# Transforming Shame with Grief and Compassion

Shame is a core element of the neglect experience and is often deeply buried. It may be obfuscated by worldly achievement; defended against by the outward focus on others; unrecognized due to disconnection or limited self-awareness; or clouded over by substance use, compulsive behavior or some other numbing activity or explanation for hiddenness or secrecy. It may be scrambled by confusion or denial, or addled by a tangle of paradoxes or apparent ironies.

Shame by its nature is about hiding, and neglect typically results in the solitude of either abandonment, social withdrawal or both. It can readily remain hidden within this isolation, which becomes a familiar and even arguably preferable default mode. The work with shame is formidable and delicate. Shame about shame itself may be one challenge. And just below it is both anger and a well of grief that our clients may have successfully avoided for their whole lives until they get to us. Compassion and dispensing with self-blame and self-hatred are the royal road to the grief that will heal, and also facilitate the healing attachments that fuel the yearning underneath it.

Because shame is endemic to the neglect experience, we can take it as pretty much given that we will encounter it. This chapter will outline the clinical markers, both to flag the areas to work on, and also identify indicators that it is resolving. We will revisit attachment theory to interpret some of the behaviors we observe; explore the paradoxical obstacles, and address the ultimate objective of compassion, finally summarizing the treatment goals.

## EYE CONTACT

Lack of eye contact is a hallmark of shame. In effect, it is a closing off or concealing of the portal to one's essential self, one's soul. Ruth Lanius writes eloquently about it, describing her work with a war veteran who was quite aware of why he averted his eyes. "I was afraid if people could see into me, they would see the stain on my soul." With some clients, the lack of eye contact is less in their awareness, and even less in awareness, their reasons for it. When I have pointed it out carefully to some of them, they may have been surprised and not ever noticed.

Again, what enables us to time and point out thoughtfully our observation about lack of eye contact, or any behavior of the client for that matter, is being ever present to our own reactivity about them. Had I not processed the age-old meanings and projections evoked by them in my own past, I likely would have sounded harsh, impatient or critical, like a scolding parent or nagging spouse. They may simply not feel safe enough to experiment with changing their eye contact yet, which in itself may contribute to an already hefty load of shame. If we are not astutely and acutely aware of ourselves, we can both miss vital information about the client and make mistakes that set us back.

The reader may notice I am fairly liberal about revealing my mistakes and even failures. I hope that does not damage my credibility. Rather than retreat into defensiveness or shame about competence, I do this partly because this work requires great courage and humility, which are also required by "ownership" or taking responsibility. And frankly, it is all too easy to make mistakes. As noted, these clients *require* us to both do our own work and obtain regular and effective consultation. But also, because I/we want to model and teach the child of neglect that mistakes are usually not a fatal blow, especially when we develop the essential ability for repair. It is a calmer and very different world when we can walk around free of the crippling or paralyzing fear of a mis-step, mis-steps which might then further fuel the shame-machinery. I have found that the experience of rupture and repair, and a non-defensive caregiver who cares enough about the relationship to attend to it, is worth even more than having gotten it "right" in the first place. But of course, not always. (Working on our own perfectionism, and the grandiosity it connotes, is always a good idea!) All that being said, we can rely on lack of eye contact as a shame marker that flags for us a painful, private story. In the case of Jackie, whom we met in Chapter 2, it went all the way back to a sad and lonely child, feeling desperately alone, rejected and afraid as she watched her body balloon up in a way that just elicited more rejection and loneliness.

Around the same time period I first worked with Jackie, I met Irv, who kept his eyes closed much of the time when he was talking to me. Similarly, having not yet done my own personal excavation, I felt annoyed and disrespected, disconnected. And I heard myself slipping into judgment, silently fighting against allegations of "laziness" lack of discipline, lack of motivation. Ugh. I hated having such thoughts. These were the very criticisms, accusations and condemnation, I later learned, that he daily heard from his busy, over-achieving, grossly neglectful parents. At that time, it was hard for me to believe him that it "hurt" his eyes to keep them open and look at me.

We now know from Lanius' research that this is actually highly plausible. Lanius, using neuroimaging technology, has extensively and systematically studied shame and eye contact in her Ottawa Ontario lab, and collected data both in the psychological and the anatomical aspects. What her trauma and neglect clients report, is that they have tremendous apprehension or fear about being seen, as if their core integral "badness" or worthlessness will be exposed and visible. Or perhaps the parents' rejection, hatred or narcissism will be defied or antagonized by the child's being seen. No surprise there. What I found enlightening and helpful was the physiology.

Because the eyes are known for being a window into the character of the other, and for calculating the other's emotions and intentions, they become an avenue of assessing safety. We all initially default to the eyes, to make a first evaluation. And for all of us, traumatized or not, there is an initial assessment for danger versus safety. If the coast is clear, the social engagement area of the cortex takes over. Lanius' neuroimaging scans showed that in the brains of survivors of trauma and neglect, who generally operate from a *baseline* level of fear, eye contact activated the reptilian, most primitive fear center, which remained activated, rather than progressing on to social engagement It is highly plausible that physical pain can accompany such activation. Most typically, however, survivors experience the fear reaction as discomfort, and avoidance becomes so reflexive, that they are not aware of it at all.

By contrast, non-traumatized controls', higher brain areas of social engagement were activated, and higher levels of oxytocin, the hormone of connection, were associated with eye contact. For the non-traumatized, eye contact can be a pleasurable conduit of relatedness. I had never much thought in this way, for example, about infants' delight in the simple game of "peek-a-boo."

Lanius' lab used virtual images to simulate the eye contact, inanimate avatars comparing the brains' response to direct gaze and averted gaze in sets of traumatized v non-traumatized subjects. As a treatment, she assigned trauma and neglect clients to practice with beloved and trusted pets. Both Jackie and Irv, had dearly loved dogs with whom they could well have practiced. I chose to make use of the therapeutic relationship, hoping to increase and enhance the safety between us.

Over time, and significant work on all our parts, I was able to verbally address the eye contact with both Jackie and Irv. With both, we became able to cautiously, rather peek-a boo-like, experiment with it. They were able to increasingly express both the fear and the shame of being visible, and later still, the isolation that had been both of their existence.

I have since also learned that just as addressing the shame more directly, i.e. explicitly targeting the emotional experience, naturally and spontaneously will alter the eye contact, The inverse is also true. As we target the eye contact, the emotional experience and possibly even the story, become both more accessible and more resolvable. So somatic targeting of eye contact can be a vehicle for commencing with the delicate work with shame.

## THE LONG PANDEMIC MONTHS FORCED US ALL TO WORK REMOTELY, AND I FOUND

Myself, as we all did, for the first time, seeing my clients on a computer screen. I for one, never dreamed I might be working this way. The often accursed, imprecise electronic medium can make it a technological challenge to precisely synchronize or align our eyes. Sometimes an irregularity of timing, other times camera angle, can leave me feeling a little "Picasso-like" with fractured or misdirected gaze. For some neglect clients, however, the remote medium, with all its foibles, has provided a safer venue to experiment or even progress with eye contact. In some cases, working the eye contact edge was intentional.

Aaron and Maureen whom we met in Chapter 7, consciously took advantage of the Zoom sessions to work with eye contact. Maureen loved facing Aaron and staring into his big brown eyes. Aaron found he could tolerate and get used to that better, if they both faced forward and made eye contact via the screen. So, our Zoom sessions actually advanced them with their eye contact discrepancy "deal." In other cases, the Zoom progress with eye contact, was one of the many unintended, unexpected, often idiosyncratic blessings of challenging times. It just appeared on its own, like a volunteer plant.

Understanding eye contact and its meanings made a huge difference in the difficult work with Ralph and Suzanne, a couple who came to me much more recently. Eye contact regularly and loudly intruded, in both content and process into our sessions as a soon predictable and wily disruption. It made its stormy appearance, literally right from our first session. Fortunately, by then I could make a better guess, at what the lack of eye contact might both mean *to* each of them, and also what it might signify *about.* each of them. The working hypotheses, admittedly "educated guess" work, lent much needed support as I strove to steady myself in their whirlwind of conflict.

## WINDOW ON NEGLECT

Ralph deflected and rejected the characterization of himself as neglected, and his family as anything but ideal, and therefore "untouchable." He did not want to talk about his childhood. He was not "antitherapy," per se, but viewed himself as logical and rational to a fault, and he did not see himself as someone who "needed" it. All he really wanted was for his despair to be known and heard. So even though he had all the hallmarks of neglect, my task was to just unobtrusively use what I know and honor his wish. Sometimes that is what we are left with, and the world of non-verbal information we are provided with. He wanted to shout from the rooftops about his misery and agonizing pain. He could not articulate what he was so catastrophically unhappy about, and I had no articulated background about this extraordinarily intelligent and similarly exceptionally professionally successful man, except what I slowly began to learn from their recurring volatile blitzkrieg about eye contact.

Ralph spoke slowly, haltingly and with long pauses. Clearly (to me), he was full of emotions, he had simply never learned a language to express them, and no one had ever wanted to hear them. He had explicitly told me he had little use for me, on more than a few occasions, and was highly doubtful that I had anything remotely helpful to offer. He was overtly disrespectful even bordering on offensive toward me I could see that the one clearest, maybe only acceptable way I could be of some minimal use to this ferociously self-reliant man, was to provide and protect the time and space for him to find his words and his emotions.

Much of the time when he talked with Suzanne and even more when she talked to him, at least in our therapy, Ralph's eyes were averted or closed. Invariably as he was elaborating a thought or articulation of some emotion, Suzanne would abruptly and sharply burst in on a pause in his words, with "Ralph! Please look at me when we're talking! You *never* look me in the eyes." And Suzanne, being a woman of many words, and great facility in speaking, would elaborate at length about this, which to Ralph felt like an unending hammering. Often, I felt like a traffic cop, or better yet a boxing referee.

After the interruptions, Ralph would collapse, clam up, and the discussion was over. He would withdraw, sometimes for days, which left her even more angry and critical. Ralph provided a spectacular and lavish lifestyle for Suzanne. He was a responsible and faithful husband, a good dad, a decent citizen of the world. He wanted to hear any mention of any of that. Suzanne would be baffled, angry and lonely; and more critical. Why did he make such a big deal about eye contact? It was a categorically "reasonable" and "healthy" request. All of her friends agreed with her. (Of course, Suzanne had her own story, but we limit ourselves to the study of Ralph.)

What Suzanne failed to understand, was that Ralph's complaint was not only about eye contact but more about criticism. He had, as do many or most children of neglect, a hypersensitive nose for criticism; which readily translated to rejection; and part of the endless quest to answer the unanswerable "why" of being unwanted. His eyes both protected and hinted at this deep grief and pain. He appeared to be quite impenetrable to my efforts, except quieting Suzanne long enough that he could voice what he was able to, which meant and achieved more than I realized. Someone was looking out for him, seeing and hearing him. But he had no words for it, so we had to wait.

One day, Ralph took out his phone to launch Spotify and played us a song. I had not ever heard it before, and I did not recognize the name of the performer. And now I remember neither, but I absolutely remember the moment. It was a soft, quiet feminine voice and guitar, in the style of folk music of the 1960s and 1970s. It was a love song, but more than that, it was about gratitude, appreciation and acceptance. It seemed to be about being seen and heard, cherished for who one is. And as we listened to the song, Ralph dissolved into convulsive tears for a long time.

Ralph never explicitly let me know what his deep, protracted shame was about. A man so accomplished and wealthy, he was ashamed of his shame. He saw himself as ungrateful and even more "bad," for feeling bad. He was ashamed of his need for Suzanne, his lonely craving for her love and her touch, for feeling wanted by her. And her seemingly unending criticism felt like a looping cycle of rejection. Only extreme reactions to feeling unheard and unseen, unacceptable as he was, and criticized, and what he experienced as a poverty of recognition and appreciation of his goodness, offered the window into his desolate history.

The song brought him to compassion. It named and opened his heart to the missing experience, and he was able to bring it into the room. Suzanne felt it too, we all did. From that point, the tension quieted. The change was subtle and steady, but he seemed to become gentler, with himself and ultimately with Suzanne.

Sometimes sensory experience is the needed key to unlock emotion and compassion, if not yet language. The moment was reminiscent of Stephen Porges' early work with autistic children at the turn of the 20th century. He then called it the Listening Project, and had the children daily listen to music digitally remastered to simulate tonal frequencies of a mother's voice. I don't know whatever happened with that work or that approach, but it fascinated and made sense to me at the time, and I never forgot about it. And I know I always seem to have a song in my head, and sometimes they serve me with these clients.

Ralph's ambivalence about therapy, however, never stopped. It was not only shame about needing help but also it continued to feel too dangerous and just too ego-dystonic to need another person, a "stranger" like me. When he decided he was quitting therapy, he was no longer afraid of Suzanne's reaction. He no longer felt so intrinsically "bad," and no longer felt compelled to accommodate the other, and do whatever the other desired.

When they left, I found myself feeling relieved. I was worn out from the devaluation and unending criticism of me. These were highly uncharacteristic feelings for this die hard sold-out-concerts girl. I had to take note of them. They sounded a little too much like Ralph. Had Ralph and Suzanne stayed in therapy with me, those feelings inside of me would have inspired me to wonder if he had decided to leave Suzanne, his growing self-acceptance feeling too dissonant with what he experienced as her chronic rejection, too hard for him to tolerate, or just not interesting anymore.

Sometimes the child of neglect can't stay the course, for whatever reason. We have to manage our own shame about that, or whatever our feelings might be. I like to think that although Ralph did not allow me to give him much, rather forcefully protecting the space for him to be seen and heard; explicitly structuring time for both Ralph and Suzanne to express their feelings, loosened his self-hatred and sense of worthlessness. He became a little more confident, kept his eyes a little more open and sat a little taller. And maybe that contributed to what seemed like the watershed, of the song.

As a young runner, I was always rather intrigued by the relay events. They were tailor-made for a child of neglect. One is part of something larger, but runs alone, only making contact when the baton is passed and the team mate takes over. Sometimes our work with these clients is rather like that. We do our best at our stint and pass the baton to some unknown team mate. No shame in that!


## SHAME ABOUT NOT KNOWING

Sometimes the shame will be about not knowing. Knowing it all, figuring it out, or figuring out *how* to figure it out, all become means of survival in a world where there is no one there to teach a child how the world works, or how fundamentals of life and social life, are done. Sometimes the child of neglect discovers fairly ingenious ways. My father, when he stowed away on a ship at age 17, to escape the Shanghai ghetto, called it "stealing with his eyes," when he "learned" how to cook in the maritime kitchen. Not being able to figure it out, or simply not knowing or having skills that everyone else seems to, or "should," can be a point not only of fear and disorientation but also shame. "What is *wrong* with *me*? Everyone else seems to know what to do!" Especially regarding social life.

The child of neglect may be ashamed of how few relationships they have had in their lives, they may be ashamed of how many. Some have combatted their shame by notching the bed post, the numbers meaning they are desirable, and "not so bad," to others it may mean they are *very* bad, depending on their moral and religious training. We may be asked to be the arbiter, or at least some sort of teacher, or confessor. Or with luck, we may become the safe resource for information that will help them with their lives. That is our hope.

Now that we have the internet, there is a limitless supply of answers, many of them sounding quite authoritative. The client may have found and embraced answers, and be proud of their resourcefulness. Some that horrify us, or seem incompatible with what we are trying to do. We must go very gently, and if possible, if they will receive it, be empathic toward the child who was not taught, and has suffered such loneliness (and ignorance) as a result.

We must be mindful of our own biases and blind spots. I had one client as she was about to turn thirty years old, sink into a bout of profound shame and loss, that the decade of her twenties had passed her by and would not be back. Due to her "ignorance," or whatever the "shortcoming" she had had about relationships, the ages that are supposed to be so much fun, now were gone. My twenties were a nightmare, and my life only got better in my thirties, forties and fifties and now sixties. But that would have been of no use to her, in her shame. Letting her rant until the rant had taken its course, brought her to the pain and grief, and the emergent awareness that it was not her "fault." That is the shift we want, whenever possible, to help to facilitate. Had I stayed with the rational, what she was sure she "knew" it would have been a squandered opportunity.

My client, Holly was one of the many, deeply embarrassed about knowing so little about the relational world. She was mortified about how badly she had bungled a relationship with a man she had truly loved. When early in their relationship he made a cross country pilgrimage to spend time specifically with her, she had no idea of the niceties of how to make him feel welcome and special. She did not pick him up from the airport, but gave him the complicated instructions about how to get to her home by public transportation; she did not buy any groceries or find out what he might like; or make any plans on the basis of what she knew about his tastes and preferences. In fact, she mostly went about her usual routines and failed to register his disappointment and discomfort. When he precipitously left and flew home, halfway through their planned visit, she was devastated. And racked with shame about being so clueless about what went wrong. Granted he had not spoken up either. But she simply treated him the way she knew, which of course was just as she had always been treated, and went about her life much as she always did. She did not register that understandably, he felt as if his visit, and he himself, did not matter. But Holly had not seen this, because not mattering was just all so "normal" to her.

From a painstaking and careful "post mortem" we systematically reviewed the visit, and the subsequent end of that relationship, a process that took us a number of painful months. And we wrangled a bit about the pace. On one hand, she could not wait to unpack it all, brimming and desperate as she was to "get it all out." And although venting was a great relief to her, she simultaneously felt increasingly horrified and deeply ashamed to reveal her poverty of relatedness, and the knowledge or ability to achieve it.

*The therapist must carefully regulate the pacing of shame disclosure,* just as we carefully regulate the pacing of any trauma work. Especially, as with Holly, I did not yet know her well and did not yet have a sense of her window of tolerance. If we don't watch our speed, as Peter Levine warns, the system explodes. "Slow always wins," says he. It was a long time, and largely due to the magnitude of the lost relationship, before Holly became able to explore underneath the shame, the loss of connection and relatedness of her whole life, that would add up to her knowing so little about the relationship world. It was much longer still before she was able to absolve herself of blame for all she did not know. But the work was deep and transformative.

It may be a long time before these clients can tolerate becoming aware of just how much they don't know. That would mean taking a hard look at how their family did or did not function; how they were left alone to glean what they could, and guess based on intuition, and the often-gross paucity or misinformation from movies, television (and porn). Earning sufficient trust, so the child of neglect will have the confidence and the humility to ask is, one of our painstaking clinical challenges. And given survival meaning attributed to depending on their own answers, timing is critical also on this, so as not to offend or threaten by the appearance of taking away or undermining a lifeline-like defense.

Holly was very concerned that I not "go too light on her." She felt an urgent eagerness to learn from and not repeat her mistakes. She kept asking me if I was holding out on her, almost as if she deserved to be punished. And sometimes the belief that punishment is in order is a considerable obstacle, if in fact what the shame is telling them, is "I'm bad," and most especially if they adhere to the age-old truism "My parents did the best they could." Yet the ultra-sensitivity to criticism is never far. It was a fine line to find with Holly to give her enough information to satisfy her, without "beating her up."

It was also useful to Holly to know more about what would go on in more "related" families; what those kids would learn that she didn't. Holly's household never had guests, let alone houseguests who stayed overnight. She knew nothing about that, or about disrupting one's usual daily routine, perhaps buying and preparing different foods, finding out tastes, planning schedules, big and little things that might make a person feel cared for. They were just foreign to her Hearing that those, would be things that kids would learn, either by being explicitly taught, or learn by experience, by being a participant, was helpful to her. The accompanying sadness about her deprivation took longer.

## SHAME TO PROTECT TRAUMATIZED PARENTS

Holly could see that a young, single mom, abandoned by a brutal, irresponsible man with little Holly as an infant; grappling with poverty, racism, and all the responsibilities of a child, a household and a job, she would rather hate *herself* than hold a critical view of her mom. Shame was a way of protecting the image of the best attachment figure she knew, and perhaps hang on to the shred of illusion (or reality) that she had in fact been wanted and loved, that her mother just "couldn't help it." For a while she wrestled with what seemed irreconcilable to her. Was her mother clueless, narcissistic and neglectful? Or simply "handicapped?" or too deprived herself? Jackie angrily struggled with the same thing. "Was it intentional, her completely ignoring me, letting me twist in the wind?" It was a revelation to both Jackie and Holly, they could feel both ways: compassion for the mother, and outrage about her failings, which were real and painful, and tremendously costly.

The intergenerational transmission of trauma creates this paradox. Traumatized parents may readily repeat what was done to them, or simply go unconscious about how they affect their children. It took me decades to integrate and make peace with the seemingly warring flashing images of my mother as a little terrified girl sitting alone on cold, clattering train barreling off into a dark night; and my own being left alone. About both being true. Holly was angry thinking, "But she never did any work on herself! To make the chain of trauma stop!" And another wave of anger.

The existential balancing act is a profound process. Over time, Holly's anger and despair about her profound neglect and loneliness, and all the lost years made sense and were not something to be ashamed of or hide, were neither "exaggerated or indulgent complaints" nor a statement about her worth. Her mother had suffered too. Feeling angry at her mother's failings was not a failure on her part. And ultimately when she was able to hold both and accept her own feelings, she felt less shame and her anger with both her mother and herself, softened. Shame gradually waned.

Jackie did feel shame as well about the lost years and the wasted life, all the things she had never done as she had spent years hiding in a life of work, and with her "head in the refrigerator." After a long time, she made a deep connection with me. Her eye contact was steady and she could even tell me that she felt my care for her. She could grieve the lost time, and also feel profound gratitude that even though she was in her 50s she was truly beginning to enjoy her life and discover what she might like to do besides work, she made new friends who loved her, and her shame evolved beyond compassion into a blooming, incredulous gratitude.

## "IS THIS 'SELF PITY' INDULGENT?"

Another hurdle along the way, or conundrum, is the seeming duality between grief and "wallowing." In a world devoid of feelings, or where it is difficult to identify what could be so wrong, grief itself may be a point of shame. Unentitled to complain as "there is '*nothing*' to complain about," sorrow may seem to be a narcissistic ego-alien indulgence or a waste of time. Or simply rationalized away. "My brother had it a whole lot worse!" We must be patient with as long as it might take before it becomes acceptable to acknowledge or feel the pain. For Holly it seemed to arise from the neurofeedback to realize that "my brother had it bad for sure. But neglect is not visible, it is about what did not happen so it may appear less scarring.

But it is still very deeply damaging." As she actually came to accept the reframe of her story, in effect construct the narrative, what followed was great relief, and a solid identification with it. Much shame dissolves with that. Their unhappiness is not unfounded or indulgent, it is not their innate worthlessness or badness. The discovery "I do have a story" and the ability to tell it, they feel less alone and categorically less ashamed.

## THE POSTURE OF SHAME

Another reliable indicator of shame, well documented by Ekman is a recognizable body organization. It consists of collapse and a body pulled back into itself. It is a graphic depiction of withdrawal, another language of the unexpressed story, like a crying out from a "secret" hiding place. Holly was horrified to catch a glimpse of her profile in the mirror and see how hunched forward she was. "I look like an old woman! An old witch!" she gasped. She went to YouTube and looked for physical therapy to improve her posture, without even knowing about its correlation to shame. She only knew how ashamed it made her feel to suddenly see that image of herself. As she found herself more upright, she felt taller, and the larger shame did not disappear, but became more accessible to speak about.

Shame is categorically difficult to verbalize about, partly because of the embarrassment that surrounds the feeling itself, but also because its meaning and function are all about hiding, so it is paradoxical to speak about it, to come out of hiding to talk about hiding. Because for many it simply feels like an unspeakable somatic and emotional wash, words often elude. When Holly sank into her shame, she really only had one word, a loudly resounding Greek chorus of "stupid, stupid, stupid, stupid, stupid …" Achingly painful to listen to, and certainly not helpful to us to allow.

Working somatically was a safer and more adaptive entrée. A readily available explicit shame measuring "tool," the "Shame Measurement Scale" can be freely found and accessed. It consists of both stick figures portraying different postural forms and text questionnaires about shame. Any of the major somatic trauma therapy approaches will have protocols for addressing shame directly through the posture, Frank Corrigan has elaborated a particularly elegant and powerful protocol that combines his own Deep Brain Reorienting with the Alexander

Method which is a long-established somatic therapy. Any of these approaches might make the difficult work with shame, more bearable.

## SUMMING UP AND WHAT TO DO

- Because shame is rooted in not wanting to be seen, it is of course challenging to uncover and address. It often lacks words and even conscious awareness. Self-hatred, self-doubt, and an all-around negative self-view are such long-held assumptions or facts of life, that it may seem there is really nothing to talk about. Like ambient air or a familiar background noise, awareness of its grip eludes.

- When available, childhood photos may illustrate both the hiding and the sadness of the child, and both can become visible. These portrayals may both elucidate and elicit memory of hiding as well as possibly grief and compassion. Of course, in the case of neglect, it is quite possible that nobody bothered taking photos of the child, which is also telling.

- When childhood photos are not available, experiment with visualization of a child, or I might recommend they watch the Still Face or Strange Situation videos available online, which often elicit shame, grief and compassion.

- If the client has children, I will ask to see photos of their own child, which may evoke feelings or memory through the contrast, or fear and shame about their own mistakes; and about passing shame and trauma on via the intergenerational chain.

- With couples, a powerful practice can be to experiment with gazing, each placing one hand on the other partner's heart, quietly and slowly breathing together, holding the eye contact for just a few seconds at first, and seeing what they might notice. Besides being for many a powerful and safe intimate moment, it can be helpful with shame.

- When no partner is available, or when a human partner or practice-mate may be too threatening, Lanius will have clients experiment with eye contact, with a safe animal friend. Many children of neglect have non-human friends who are their most loved and intimate relationships, (and are very devoted to animal-related humanitarian causes).

- Somatic work with body posture, opening up the somatic hiding place.
- As ever being the safe and present attachment figure, available to sensitively, and patiently answer questions and provide some of that normalizing vital information they never got, especially about relationship and sexuality.
- Provide the compassion until they can.
- We can as good as assume that shame will be an expectable accompaniment to childhood neglect. Identifiable markers of shame are: lack of eye contact; hypersensitivity to what they perceive as criticism; an almost instantaneous translation/ interpretation of criticism as rejection; tendency toward isolation and hiding; a distinct body organization of collapse and withdrawal, stooped forward, downcast eyes, and the pulled-back heart protected by rolled forward neck and shoulders.
- Children being self-referential, will reflexively and immediately default to an explanation that the neglect was due to something endemic to themselves, and fill in the blank in their own unique way. That manifestation or symptom of their worthless or hateful nature may coagulate into what they think of as the "presenting problem," such as Jackie's weight. Or it may be a largely unconscious shadow they carry inside, that impels them to isolate and hide.
- The therapist staying aware of it and anticipating shame may help with the difficulties of bringing it forward.
- Shame may also be a way of protecting or defending against some impulse to attack or blame the parent.
- Any moment of compassion the therapist can offer counts and helps. Shame may portend one of our more rocky roads.

## BIBLIOGRAPHY

Corrigan, Frank M., and Jessica Christie-Sands. "An Innate Brainstem Self-Other System Involving Orienting, Affective Responding, and Polyvalent Relational Seeking: Some Clinical Implications for a 'Deep Brain Reorienting' Trauma Psychotherapy Approach." *Medical Hypotheses* 136, no. 109502 (March 2020). https://doi.org/10.1016/j.mehy.2019.109502.

Ekman, Paul. *Emotions Revealed: Recognizing Faces and Feelings to Improve Communication and Emotional Life.* Revised ed. New York: Owl Books, 2003.

Frewen, Paul A., and Ruth A. Lanius. *Healing the Traumatized Self: Consciousness, Neuroscience, Treatment.* Norton Series on Interpersonal Neurobiology. New York: W. W. Norton, 2015.

Levine, Peter A. *In an Unspoken Voice: How the Body Releases Trauma and Restores Goodness.* Berkeley, California: North Atlantic Books, 2010.

Levine, Peter A. *Trauma and Memory: Brain and Body in a Search for the Living Past; A Practical Guide for Understanding and Working With Traumatic Memory.* Berkeley, California: North Atlantic Books, 2015.

Porges, Stephen W., Katherine E. Bono, Mary Anne Ullery, Olga Bazhenova, Andreina Castillo, Elgiz Bal, and Keith Scott. "Listening to Music Improves Language Skills in Children Prenatally Exposed to Cocaine." *Music and Medicine* 10, no. 3 (July 2018): 121–129. http://dx.doi.org/10.47513/mmd.v10i3.636.

Schwarz, Lisa, Frank Corrigan, Alastair M. Hull, and Rajiv Raju. *The Comprehensive Resource Model: Effective Therapeutic Techniques for the Healing of Complex Trauma.* Explorations in Mental Health. New York: Routledge, 2017.

Steuwe, Carolin, Judith K. Daniels, Paul A. Frewen, Maria Densmore, Sebastian Pannasch, Thomas Beblo, Jeffrey Reiss, and Ruth A. Lanius. "Effect of Direct Eye Contact in PTSD Related to Interpersonal Trauma: An fMRI Study of Activation of an Innate Alarm System." *Social Cognitive and Affective Neuroscience* 9, no. 1 (January 2014): 88–97. https://doi.org/10.1093/scan/nss105.

Vineyard, Missy. *How You Stand, How You Move, How You Live: Learning the Alexander Technique to Explore Your Mind-Body Connection and Achieve Self-Mastery.* New York: Marlowe and Company, 2007.

Chapter **9**

# GPS

This chapter is intended to serve as a snapshot, to summarize, review and organize all the many elements we have traversed, into a coherent, sequential road map. Just as our goal is to have the client leave with a knowable, comprehensible and believable continuous life story to tell and re-tell, I want the reader to close the covers of this book, with a clear and practical sense of direction and trajectory. Like all psychotherapy, we cannot hope to prescribe a single recipe for all, but a prototype perhaps. Like a Global Positioning System, the intent is to orient, to roughly position us in space. Where possible, I will try to include a bit of neurobiology, partly because I find it so fascinating, and partly because often our clients find it reassuring and perhaps even vindicating, that something they may have been mortally ashamed of, is shared with everyone else and often even other mammals. That, however, will come more in the following chapter about methodologies that highlight the brain more centrally.

Finally, where possible, I again will mention here, some lessons learned the hard way, so that my missteps will serve us all. Safe, knowledgeable and reliable consultation is crucially necessary, and as I am fond of saying, "Find the best consultation money can buy, tell them *everything*, and do what you're told!" Any success I have ever had, is rooted in that.

**"LOST IN SPACE"**

In the late 1990s, I remember a little flurry of reports of whopping PTSD reactions of surgery patients, insufficiently anesthetized, who partially woke up during their surgeries. Conscious enough to hear the horrific sounds of cutting flesh, and conversations among the medical practitioners not intended for their ears; and to feel searing, excruciating pain. But medicated enough to be locked in, immobility and silence. Unable to get the attention of the busy surgery team, by speech or gesture, they had no choice but to helplessly endure. These were daunting clients to treat. If they appeared in therapy at all, they were understandably hesitant to trust a caregiver and lacked sharp or coherent memory of the event, so their "story" was rather a cloudy emotional blur.

In 2010, I was particularly gripped by the news of a group of 32 Chilean miners trapped 5 miles underground when the mine collapsed. For 69 days they helplessly waited, with no one knowing where they were, unable to communicate or take any purposeful action on their own behalf. Thankfully they were all excavated alive, but the story compelled me. It was another example, like the surgery patients, dramatically illustrating the core tasks in working with neglect: to *sow and cultivate voice and agency*. By voice we mean the ability to speak, both in articulating need and want: their existence, and ultimately their story; and participating as equals in present time relationship. By agency we mean to emerge from the mode of powerless waiting, into strength, confidence and impulse for purposeful interpersonal action. These again, are our most fundamental objectives.

Jackie by now is well known to us. As we know, she came to therapy ostensibly due to an unremitting weight issue, and an even more unremitting obsession about it. The worst of her trauma, she later came to understand, was the incomprehensible reality that as the pounds conspicuously piled on, no one, saw or intervened with a helping hand. "No one said a word. It was as if I were drowning while all of my most trusted others continued happily sunbathing on the shore." She added, "I don't get it. Fat people, young or old, are unbearably conspicuously visible. We get stared at, even ogled. How can it be that at the same time, we can be so completely invisible?" The failure to elicit attention or care, in any way that originated with herself, spawned the earliest seeds or spores of worthlessness, powerlessness and passivity. How wildly they proliferate! These are what are most essential to repair.

Jackie was not aware of anger or frustration. Weight was the persistent, presenting issue. This is generally the case. Rarely does a client come to therapy to work on neglect, or developmental trauma. Like Jackie, they believe they are coming to work on a glaring symptom: a drug history, failed relationships, depression, which is certainly not untrue. It is unlikely to be convincing, however, and not necessary to disabuse them of their own idea of the most important reason why they have come. As ever to *meet them where they are.*

## FIRST OBSTACLES

As we have seen in detail, emotions are not only a foreign language but often a nuisance or even pain to be avoided. The inherent value of emotion is a hard sell at best. If they have not been in therapy before, our clients often arrive *thinking* they want an explanation of how this is supposed to work; or as in Jackie's case, how is this going to be different from her previous long drawn out and expensive "waste of time" therapy experiences. What will we *do*? It probably won't make sense, however. Said one middle-aged man, annoyed and humiliated, when I made the mistake of answering the question with a longwinded explanation of about Attachment Theory "So you're telling me I'm a two-year-old!" He imagined I would or was manipulating him into being angry at his mother. He loudly and immediately let me know, "I feel condescended to and disrespected. Actually, I'm angry at *you*!" We need to be cautious about their questions; inquire and work at hearing what they really want to know, if anything really. It may be that what they are testing for is some sort of safety. They don't know really what question they might ask that would answer that. Most likely what is really underneath their questions, is "I'm afraid there is no help for me." Or "I'm afraid one more caregiver will fail me." They may or may not be open to exploring that. And if they arrive with a dustbin of failed past therapies, which some do, we must be sufficiently grounded and have enough support to weather their ambivalent mistrust (which may feel rather insulting at times!).

Jackie, whose default was more to numbing and depression, had a seemingly mechanical model of getting "fixed," almost imagining that the therapist had some sort of magical armamentarium for reaching in and moving things around, so as to rearrange or extract her dysfunctions. She brought somewhat of that misconception to her curiosity about EMDR, wondering when I would bring it on, and if *it* would work. It was as if the modality or the therapist would work, not she herself, or us as a team. And of course, if it was not the modality or technique that succeeded or failed, it was the all-powerful other, the therapist. Jackie had had nothing but disappointments beginning with both of her parents, and really everyone since. So, the questioning, "how will you be different?" "What is wrong with me?" or the perennial "why?" "Why am I so unhappy?" "Why do these things keep happening to me?" may have a kind of desperation and urgency. Rather than getting caught in answering the unanswerable question, which is really "Can I trust you?" we must be present and begin to get the picture of a long history void of help and trust. We begin to try and construct a story out of emptiness. If anything, we can validate their doubt. "Of course, it would be a tall order to trust me or any other caregiver or person in 'authority.' I will do my utmost to *earn* your trust."

Early on when I first started working with these clients, a signature of neglect showed itself to be "I don't know what to do." Or "there's nothing I can do," accompanied by the now familiar profound, abiding, shrugging hopeless helplessness. They had never had an impact, they had had no power over when or if ever there would be any attention or connection for them. I have since learned that the dorsolateral prefrontal cortex, the brain area that is stimulated by the mother-infant gaze, in a secure attachment, is also related to agency and purposeful action. The underdevelopment of that area will result in a default to freeze and collapse. And where Jackie was a powerful, effective and highly respected professional at work, in the interpersonal, she would evaporate. It wasn't even on her radar to work on that. She believed that to be pointless; it was somewhere in her DNA, and she would always be alone. There was nothing she could do.

Perhaps paradoxically, another challenge for the therapist, as noted, is the fierce conviction that they *know*. Fierce because growing up essentially alone, they had no choice. It was survival to find their own answers because there was nowhere else to turn. On one hand *we*, as the caregiver, expert or "grown-up" are supposed to know. On the other, they are convinced that they know best, they *must*. They may even try to run the therapy. They do not dare imagine that we might know more, or taking a chance on what we know. So even though Jackie thought she was coming to try EMDR, she was in no hurry to relinquish control into my unknown hands, but also into the grips of an unknown medium.

Challenging, or "taking away" what they think they know, may feel to the child of neglect, like cutting them off from a lifeline, and leaving them lurching alone in a roiling sea. Terrifying and unforgivable. This ferocious and insistent knowing ironically persists alongside the helpless refrain of "I don't know." The fact is, when there is no one to push up against, there is no way to know, what they know and what they don't know. And there is no opportunity to individuate and experience a distinct existence. Like a shape shifting amoeba, searching for a boundary, there is no self.

Jackie's confusion about the parameter of her body was a fitting metaphor. Similarly, Alison who had struggled with profound body dysmorphia and recurring bouts of anorexia, would spend hours going from store to store, trying on clothes. She never bought anything, but rather combed the racks, looking to the elusive numbers on the labels to answer the unending question about her size. She couldn't figure it out. Perhaps the fact that she could put on the lowest numbered size and it fit her, meant she was not fat? But she couldn't be sure. After all, the sizes weren't standard, the fancier brands showing lower numbers for larger sizes, the European sizes … It all left her with her head spinning, and still no answers. She would slink away ashamed, embarrassed to leave the dressing rooms, a littered mess of expensive garments, for the unwitting salesperson to clean up. Invariably she fled as confused as before, and no doubt, not thin enough.

As a young therapist, I worried and wobbled about whether new clients would "stick." They might express their ambivalence verbally, or in lateness, cancellations or persistent despair. Once again, the therapist must have the resilience, strength and support to endure this. This is where long bicycle rides, rhythmic and drawn out stirring of the cheese vat, or whatever are your regulating practices would be; my own personal therapy and neurofeedback; and of course, the "best consultation money can buy" are immeasurably valuable. This is hard work.

When these clients do stay the course, having hung in there together through the uncertainty, will be a uniquely meaningful part of our history together, like war veterans emerging alive together from the trenches. Take as given that the "real" main reason they are with us is their profound and painful challenge around relatedness. They may be aware of their loneliness, or that their relationships are unstable, volatile, unrewarding, short lived, even non-existent; or they may simply feel some undefined sense of ennui. I hold the working hypothesis that the core injury is what Frank Corrigan has so aptly named "attachment shock" until I learn otherwise. It is indeed a shock, when the evolutionary birthright of a safe and sustaining other, to shepherd us through at least those early years, Presumptuous as this may sound, to think we know, it has served me well.

As therapists, we must know our own specific vulnerabilities, and be able or sufficiently supported to tolerate the devaluation. Again, when we do "make it" the memory and the relationship will be deep and precious. Again, the essential task of the therapist is to be present, to listen and mirror, to remember, and to convey to the client that they are accurately seen. This is not all that is required of us, but it is foundational. I can't emphasize it enough.

## CONSTRUCTING THE STORY

How do we formulate a story out of "nothing?" out of empty space, out of deficit and absence? Especially when the clients themselves have little to tell, we must rely on other media of communication. When I first met Jim, he was a skinny young man in his late twenties. The presenting problem he brought was depression. He had his own lexicon of language which I had to attempt to learn, about his depression. It could be frustrating, seeming at times like he was attempting to be special or purposely opaque, so a psychiatrist trying to answer questions about medications, had no idea what he was talking about.

There was "the Real Thing" which was akin to being dunked in boiling oil but not allowed to die, rather endure the pain of melting flesh for intervals just long enough to stay alive and excruciatingly suffer more. Like Prometheus, chained and forced endlessly to relive the same mortal agony. There was also the "black" variety a notch less searing, which seemed to translate to an explosive rage. And then there was his baseline, which anyone else would have called acute clinical depression, but to him was just an ordinary day. On those days, sitting with him was as if he were under water with a mouth full of marbles while I attempted to read his lips through the blur and bubbles of muddy slush. He was quite dissociated. I was challenged to translate his metaphors into emotional or body states that I could comprehend. What I learned to do was imagine the vulnerability of an infant's body and primitive emotional states. An infant left alone; an infant looking up into an expressionless, lost, fearful or angry face. What would be the felt experience of that tiny being?

That bundle of writhing nerve endings and needs? I found myself often defaulting to such imagery, most often unbidden. And to be honest, it has often informed me, or led the hypothesis that helps me at least attempt to begin to construct the story. Of course, I must not be too attached to my own pictures. But more often than not, such a process can serve as the bridge or the stepladder out of the morass of wordless aloneness. All the somatic therapies; and even the psychodynamic approaches, teach us to be keenly aware of our own internal experience to guide or inform our work. Most definitely when in search of an unknown untold story. More than with any other client population, I rely on what I hear and see inside myself.

Jim came from a well to do and highly educated family. His father, proudly Ivy League was a successful businessman and accomplished athlete. His mother was "proper," "reasonable" and "concerned." On the rare good day when Jim showed me his genuinely funny side, he hilariously impersonated her. I had occasion to meet Jim's parents once. Mom was precisely as he portrayed her. Jim, in Dad's footsteps, was slated for the Ivy Leagues and attended one of the country's top schools, for two nightmarish years until he flunked out miserably and sank into depression, and his chosen escapes of the whole panoply of recreational drugs, heavy metal and science fiction.

Those two first Ivy League years are barely more coherent than a black stain in Jim's memory a vanishing nightmare. He ultimately found his way to and then finally graduated from a "hippie" school and moved to the Bay Area. What stood out prominently from that one visit with his parents, and what I could not forget, was how Jim's father said to me, "He's a good kid. I think he just needs help with his portfolio. I do try to help him with his portfolio." What I barely understood then because it seemed so uncanny, was that he was referring to Jim's holdings in stocks and investments, *that* was his problem. And Jim's mother, who looked rather like Julia Child without the charisma and humor, in a sensible suit and sensible pumps did not appear to disagree. Jim was quietly "under water," and I was dumbfounded. But it was infinitely useful information for me, in my data collection probe. I was later to hear more about what I came to understand as Jim's father's complete and utter obliviousness, and the narcissism, which of course eclipsed whatever shred of existence Jim might have felt he had.

One childhood story Jim did recount, was of a rare father-son activity: a mammoth mountain hike. Jim's father was quite the outdoorsman. He prided himself in having a two-digit REI (perhaps the first US recreational equipment company, established in 1938) membership number. On the day of the hike, apparently, Jim's father did not help the little five-year-old to get ready, nor did his mother, so Jim put on his sneakers with his regular thin, school socks, like he always did. As the two ascended the long miles into the chilly altitudes, Jim's feet felt increasingly frozen. When he complained, his father reproached him to "stop belly aching and soldier on." His father was an endurance athlete long before it was fashionable. He wanted his young son to toughen up as well. When they got home at the end of the long outing, Jim's feet were seriously frost bitten and he was lucky he did not lose toes. Somehow Jim did not remember his mother having had anything to say about it.

Jim did remember of course, when he was six and his older sister died precipitously. She was only a few years older than he, she had always been there. He did not understand what had happened and no one took the time to help him make sense out of it. The day of the funeral he was left at home alone. Jim's mother told him that later that day, that "God had taken Alice because she was so good." She was a little angel apparently. This was very confusing to him, and he remembered his mother crying and closing herself in her bedroom quite frequently, and for a long time. He had not ever seen her cry before, which in itself scared him. These were some of the few and far between bits and pieces of story I was able to learn directly from Jim.

## "THE INCIDENT"

Perhaps most enlightening, an epoch-making event in our history together, was what Jim came to call "the incident." This was when I made an unforgivable mistake. I agree, I made an admittedly stupid and unthinking comment. He was deliberating a personal decision and I said something on the order of "you would be a fool to do *that.*" Of course, I should not have said that, and of course, I apologized, but once the horse was out of the gate, it took off ferociously and metamorphosed into a rage that blazed uncontainable for over three years. The recent wildfires that ravaged California were pale in comparison. Jim was so incensed and outraged, that he went all over town booking consultation appointments with my colleagues to determine if it was a reportable malpractice offense, or to seek some sort of

validation, support and understanding that I had done him insuffer-
able harm, behind the closed doors. It was well beyond negligence,
and ignorance. I was terrified, wondering if he could destroy my
standing in the community. But he also would not leave the therapy
with me, or even change his multiple session per week schedule with
me. He came to them all. And he raged. He was so fierce that one day
he even kicked my chair while I was sitting in it. That was where I
drew the line. I stood up and said in no uncertain terms, "No! I will
listen to what you have to say, but violence against me or my things
will not be tolerated!" And I knew that both that some part of his story
was being blindly expressed. And most likely no one was ever strong
or present enough to really push against, let alone be contained by.

I proceeded to run all over the country consulting and training
with the best trauma experts money could buy, to help me figure out
what was going on. This was long before "trauma-informed" was a
glimmer in anyone's vocabulary, and both availability and shame
kept me from finding help near home. Clearly, Jim was in some sort
of re-enactment, he was living the unremembered experience, trying to tell me the story.

Somehow, and I have no idea how, I concluded, if I could stay
present and continue trying to understand, without becoming a victim myself, something might come of it, perhaps it would help us
reconstruct his story. It was three plus long years of relentless ven-
omous fury, three and four sessions per week. Looking back, we are
both rather incredulous, that we both hung in there, and we endured
it. How did we do it? My strategy for withstanding it and staying in it
with him, the only thing that kept me in my chair rather than sailing
(or crashing) right through the roof of my office, was to write down
everything he said, verbatim. I ended up with three huge folders,
each about three inches thick, full of notes. I still have them in the
office file cabinet, but have never even cracked one open since. It
has been twice long enough now that I could shred them, but I have
not done that either. It may have been the most razor sharp, precise
information about his childhood I would ever receive. But the lived
experience in all its blazing vividness, even more so.

As the third consecutive year slowly wound down, Jim began to
settle. It is rather a traumatic memory for me, so admittedly I do not
remember details. But what I do know is that it irreversibly changed
something for us. To this day, as his life gets better and better, and
he has cohered and healed to become a truly likable adult person,

he is now able to be and express immeasurably grateful that I stuck it out with him. He feels regret, remorse, bafflement and shame about it. But it is as if we are war comrades. We survived a battle even though we were in supposedly opposite camps at the time. Both of us are proud that we hung in there together, and he really came to trust me. As my neurofeedback consultant and angel said to me years later, "You turned him into someone you could love." And I do.

Jim's unremembered story was about being radically invisible and inaudible, and unable to communicate his pain, his need and his longing. And an epitome of despair about being viewed as "a fool" or a disappointment, or acceptable only if he did the bidding of the other. He could not yell loud enough or kick hard enough to get a response, or to exist in the mind of any other. Until now. How did I tolerate it? I can only credit my Holocaust Survivor father and his echoing words, "You should always go to sold out concerts. You'll get in."

This is a long way of saying, that often, the most reliable way of learning and re-constructing the unknown narrative, is through the therapeutic relationship: being very mindful and attuned to all that goes on there is paramount. Also, remember that the constructing of narrative is the work of the whole trajectory of the therapy. Having a mostly coherent story is one of the indicators we look for that our work is done. I might add, that thankfully we have more and powerful methodologies to help us now, than Jim and I had in those bad old days.

## SYMPTOMS

Often our neglect clients arrive with specific complaints. Because I am a relationship therapist and a sex therapist, of course, many find me through those avenues. My experience of neglect survivors in a partnership, is that most often they view the partner as pathological, and themselves as rather victim-like "endurers" or caretakers. My perennial and vociferous objection has been that the "Big T" trauma survivor gets all the blame and all the help. The neglect survivor, may be off the hook in that paradigm, but they also don't get any help, and they are invisible again. So, I am adamantly against it. It is true, that the neglect experience trains them to be endurers and caretakers, and to feel helpless to effect any other role or response in relationship. But I don't buy that that is their lot in life, nor that the partner needs to be "fixed." However, again, they are often most "comfortable" or at home in that powerless but "blameless" stance.

When we are unable to inspire a recognition of their own historical pain, and their own contribution to the difficulty, we can work at helping them discover a voice, and experience interpersonal power, as opposed to being ever at the mercy of the other. Also learning to speak about themselves and their own experience will most certainly help them to be heard. If their "caretaking" involves being a "know it all" or diagnostician, and prescriptive or judgmental in relation to the partner, they often evoke the precise opposite of what they crave, which is to feel *wanted*. It is not easy to help them to see this either. It is a wonderful surprise when they do succeed in effective self-expression, and achieving the desired outcome of actually having the partner respond by moving closer and indeed wanting them. Still, it may take a long time and many "dos-a-dos-like", forward and back defaults to the age-old behavior, before the new one sticks. *Getting a voice in relationship* as noted, is one of the fundamental tasks for the child of neglect. Advocating for this, coaching it in any way possible, and with caution against sounding patronizing or condescending, and patiently attempting to re-enforce it are part of our ongoing mission.

Addictions may be another common symptom. Alcohol and drugs can be an effective medium of escape, and may also serve as a "social lubricant" for those who feel completely ill-equipped or unfit for social life. Jim drank copiously when he first started with me, and smoked upward of two packs a day. In a desperate attempt to self-regulate, in an effort to feel alive or to feel less terror of people. Although he was at times distressed about it himself, he also fell into a habit of lying to me about it, particularly when he missed appointments from being hung over or asleep. Then he would feel terrible shame and remorse about lying to me. It also put me in the sticky bind between saying nothing, which could resemble neglect; or being the perennial nag. It became even more charged when there was a dramatic and pervasive rash of cancer in my family which he knew something about as it affected my schedule sometimes. He felt embarrassed and self-conscious about smoking, which always went along with the drinking. I don't pretend to be skilled in working with addiction nor do I care to, however, sometimes with these clients it will be part of the package. It behooves us to have good referrals and good resources to call on for when as in my case, it is not our strong suit. Just know and view it as another in the endless quest to calm or awaken an under or over-aroused nervous system, never regulated or taught to self-regulate by a reliable other.

Attention is another often encountered area of difficulty. Many survivors of childhood neglect have traumatic childhood memories of learning problems that may or may not have been labeled ADD or ADHD, depending on their elementary school era. Many of our clients come with the stories of abject terror of the reading circle, so ashamed and confused by their inability to read aloud like the other kids; hating to be exposed. Not being able to focus or concentrate in class, being bored, restless, unable to wait their turn. Many were placed on Ritalin before they knew it. Many simply went un-noticed, neglected, under-performed and had a different future than they may have, or than they may have dreamed. There may be grief work to be done around this; shame to heal, or simply understanding and self-forgiveness.

In consultation, Ruth Lanius agreed that early dorsolateral prefrontal under-activation, and the under-stimulated and therefore underdeveloped Central Executive Network, the command center of cognitive and verbal function, may account for these deficits. She also reminds us that PTSD is the only diagnosis in the book, that accounts for the *cause* of the difficulty, whatever it may be. She cautions that sometimes what is diagnosed as ADD or ADHD might be developmental trauma, and she adds that these kids may not even respond to the usually prescribed ADD medications.

Thankfully, at last "trauma-informed" is entering the mainstream vocabulary and thinking, as well as the education field. I have long been alarmed by the generation who grew up taking amphetamines, and may still be. What effect this might have on the individual and intergenerational transmission? Suffice it to say, that the complaint of attentional symptoms is a possible complaint or symptom of neglect that we must explore thoughtfully. The larger field needs to study it further, in light of developmental deficits. Treatment approaches, beginning with our own, must be curious and thorough in inquiring and understanding it, and how we treat or refer out for it. I certainly see how it can create havoc in relationship. Casting attentional deficits in the rubric of neglect, may help stimulate compassion for both the sufferer and the partner. Attentional problems certainly intersect with dissociation which is a well-known complication of both "Big T" and developmental trauma.

Often, we encounter an overlay of Big T trauma over a deeper layer of neglect. It is generally difficult for traumatic events to occur in the presence of a watchful and protective caregiver. We also know how crucial the response or non-response of the caregiver post trauma, is to the trauma's impact. Because overt traumatic events are more obvious and more likely to be at least minimally remembered (but not always!). The point here is that the underlying, early and unremembered neglect may be an even deeper injury, certainly in the area of relationship, which is usually where our clients suffer the most. Even when the trauma is particularly heinous, the under-layer of neglect may be where the most potent heartbreak and dys-regulation occurred, or at least began. Again, as it won't be remembered, we must watch and listen for it, and work with all of it.

Finally, when the client's parents had their own trauma, which so many did, our client feels they have no "right to complain." With two Holocaust survivor parents, I felt like my father simply could not be matched, and I should stop my bellyaching, just like Jim. Minimizing, shame, denial and dissociation are ready responses to parents' usually unprocessed traumatic histories. Guilt and anger may come later. I grew up hearing about "children starving in Europe" and my father going to bed hungry, as the constant reminder that I had nothing to complain about. I extrapolated from there that my suffering could not compare and that I had no right to exist. These are tough wounds to heal, which is why I have been so inspired throughout my career, to interrupt the intergenerational transmission of trauma, in all the ways we can. Helping our trauma-tized and neglected clients to stay present and protect their children. It will be healing for them, and the larger world, as well.

## NEARING COMPLETION

What are the indicators that an end might be in sight? Rosie and Steve were teachers about this. With their extreme if different, neglect histories both suffered brutally from jealousy. In both of their families, there was not enough to go around, of any vital emotional resources, or any resources really. Both were "poor little rich kids" being from fairly well to do families. Successful, well educated, attractive, intelligent, interesting- from the outside they had it all. Certainly, that was how each saw the other. Both felt significant shame about not having much else to show for their years, besides a successful career and a decent bank account. Both of their relationship histories were bleak and empty. And when they met at mid-life, as smitten as they were with each other, they suffered an agony of shameful and fearful jealousy about the past relationships of the other. Steve could not get over, how one of the characters from Rosie's relationship past was a man who was not only successful but also powerful and famous. And the relationship had spanned, off and on, years and decades of her life. The man had never been faithful or good to her, but he was a powerful famous guy who came in and out *for decades*. How could Steve compete? What would prevent him from coming back? Always eclipsed by his brother, and growing up with a narcissistic mother and absent father, Steve had long resigned himself to vanish into forgotten insignificance, coming in last. He could not believe that would not happen again.

Rosie's experience was to be of value only as a pretty doll, with the right clothes and the perfect weight, a hood ornament for her father's racecar. She could not imagine being able to compete with Steve's ex, whom although she wasn't even very kind to Steve, seemed so much more glittery, interesting and worthy.

It was a defining moment in a couple's session where again we were wrestling with this gnawingly persistent jealousy material. I said, "Rosie, tell Steve how you *felt* in relation to Bruce," the powerful famous guy. She responded "I felt nothing. He didn't see me. He didn't know who I was. All those years, he really didn't know who I was. He was big and powerful and famous. And I was an ornament. I was lonely! So alone."

I said, "Now, tell Steve how you feel with him." She turned toward him and her eyes welled up. She said with a strong voice, "With you I feel that I *exist*! I've *NEVER* felt that before. I feel joy and I feel love. And in your eyes, I can see that I do in fact exist!" This is when we know we are almost there.

## SUMMARY AND WHAT TO DO

- Initiating a relationship that will be the foundational container for our work.
- Gently identifying/introducing the experience of neglect, knowing that it may take time before an identification with it catches hold.

- Collecting data to formulate narrative, which will be ongoing.
- Beginning the work of accessing emotion. Where there is a real deficit, where often there is, relying on the body or somatic approaches to contact them.
- Being ever cognizant of shame as an ambient presence. And guilt as well.
- Finding a voice. Learning to use it, especially giving voice to emotion.
- Finding "spine," meaning the opposite of shame. The confidence and the impulse to occupy space in relationship; in effect discovering the entitlement to exist, and agency.
- All of this means creating connectivity in brain areas that failed to develop the connections to one another, that facilitates all the rest.

## BIBLIOGRAPHY

Corrigan, Frank M., and Jessica Christie-Sands. "An Innate Brainstem Self-Other System Involving Orienting, Affective Responding, and Polyvalent Relational Seeking: Some Clinical Implications for a 'Deep Brain Reorienting' Trauma Psychotherapy Approach." *Medical Hypotheses* 136, article no. 109502 (March 2020). https://doi.org/10.1016/j.mehy.2019.109502.

Illiano, Cesar. "Rescue Near for Chile Miners Trapped for Two Months." *Reuters* (October 8, 2010). https://www.reuters.com/article/us-chile-mine-rescue/rescue-near-for-chile-miners-trapped-for-2-months-idUSTRE6973I920101009.

Khalighinejad, Nima, Steven Di Costa, and Patrick Haggard. "Endogenous Action Selection Processes in Dorsolateral Prefrontal Cortex Contribute to Sense of Agency: A Meta-Analysis of tDCS Studies of 'Intentional Binding.'" *Brain Stimulation* 9, no. 3 (May 2016): 372–379. https://doi.org/10.1016/j.brs.2016.01.005.

Osterman, Janet E., and Bessel A. van der Kolk. "Awareness During Anesthesia and Posttraumatic Stress Disorder." *General Hospital Psychiatry* 20, no. 5 (September 1998): 274–281. https://doi.org/10.1016/S0163-8343(98)00035-8.

Tobar, Héctor. *Deep Down Dark: The Untold Stories of Thirty-Three Men Buried in a Chilean Mine, and the Miracle That Set Them Free.* New York: Picador, 2014.

# Chapter 10

# Beyond Words

In the quest to construct narrative out of what is often, at least partially wordless, we need a selection of access routes. Often neglect begins well before the child is verbal; and well before the cognitive brain has developed. So, the equipment to lay down "semantic" narrative-like autobiographical memory has not yet come online. Impressionistic memory fragments are unintegrated and adrift, and as we are largely dealing with *missing* experience, the work is all the more complex. If our clients' history is not fully available by cognitive and verbal means, we need more than cognitive and verbal means to work with and to reconstruct it.

Blessedly, we now have a number of recognized, effective, even increasingly evidence-based methodologies to choose between or to combine, (as well as a vast market of quick fixes and gadgetry that our clients will readily tell us about!). For each client and each therapist, there are modalities best suited to the unique skills, personalities, strengths and weaknesses of that person. In this chapter, we will review what I have come to find as the modalities most synchronous with my particularities and resources, and most congruent with the goals of our work with neglect. It will of course not be exhaustive. There is always more to read and learn, and with luck there will continue to be new and reliable data that will inform and guide us.

Many of us try out, and hone a number of selections. Some of us keep the collection open and available, others of us find a favorite and land there primarily. My experience of the last 35 years has been rather a "serial monogamy" of modalities, although each one along the way has stayed alive and continues to be an active or partial influence, even if I don't formally practice it anymore. The era of the COVID Pandemic has forced us to creatively utilize or adapt whatever factors and approaches we might have available, as we coped with "distance psychotherapy." We have seen, the more flexible and diverse our offerings the better. That is probably really always true. And because there is no shortage of bogus, novel, opportunistic or commercially driven options, as ever I recommend having solid and reliable consultation and trusted reference people to whom we can ask with confidence, "What do you think about this one?" Especially before we invest what is often considerable time and money into training and equipment.

And we will briefly visit the always relevant and all too easily overlooked, requisite of good therapist self-care, and attention to our most essential and in this work primary of instruments.

I imagine most of us have read Bessel van der Kolk's now omnipresent masterwork on trauma healing, *The Body Keeps the Score* which stolidly and obstinately refuses to budge from *The New York Times* Bestseller list for now going on seven years. It continues to be the best resource I know as both a compendium of reputable and researched methodologies useful for all types of trauma and a good explanation for why a varied approach is necessary. User-friendly, it can also be recommended to interested or skeptical clients who would like to know or understand more, before trying something unknown to them, particularly if it involves their brain! I recommend it as a comprehensive overview of, and a good introduction to a range of modalities.

I have long been goaded by a nagging motivation to speed up the work of trauma healing. I view it as a cruel injustice, and insult added to the injury, that after a lonely, vacuous, or tortured childhood, years of effort and expense are required to in effect, climb out of a hole. My now familiar clients Jackie and Jim both approached the age of 60 never having experienced the joy of rewarding partnership and love. Rosie and Steve whom we met in Chapter 9, were only discovering it now in mid-life. And Holly, who also appeared throughout the book, suffered the added loss of her childbearing years having gotten away. A recurrent theme is the tremendous and understandable grief about lost time.

The "talking cure" was once all we had. And it can be not only slow but also insufficient. Some of what we have to process must be accessed by other means. My quest has ever been to learn not only effective but also quicker safe modalities. While always also remembering the timeless sage words "The long way is the short way, and the short way is the long way." So without cutting corners, as new reliable, safe, productive and efficient approaches became available that is what I have attempted to do, and to outline here.

## KNOWLEDGEABLE AND SAFE MEDICAL BACK-UP

As noted, I entered the then nascent subfield of trauma in the early 1980s, not long after the PTSD diagnosis first appeared in the Diagnostic and Statistical Manual. The first treatment innovation to burst on the scene was Prozac, in 1988. Initially we hoped it would be a boon for PTSD sufferers. I set about putting in place a knowledgeable trauma-informed (although we did not have that term then) or at least compatible psychiatrist to whom I could refer people.

Although pharmaceuticals are rarely my "go-to" it is still worth having a solid, knowledgeable, respectful medical rearguard if one is not an MD oneself. Our healthcare system is now more complicated, so the client may have less choice. At the very least, we need trusted people to whom we can take our questions. Psych meds may sometimes be indicated or desired by developmental trauma clients. And similarly, developmental trauma both stresses and strikes the body in sometimes unusual ways. Many of our clients who have suffered "atypical" somatic symptoms have long felt disrespected or un-helped by the medical field. Jackie was repeatedly told to "just eat less and exercise more," and reached the point of feeling not only shamed but also retraumatized by the healthcare system. Another neglect survivor had a series of cycling autoimmune "attacks" from intransigent constipation to disabling migraines that were often the expression of her history, but also had an undeniable real time impact. It took us a long time to find health care people who were both familiar and patient with such symptoms.

## EMDR

The first "new" modality after Prozac that came along was EMDR (Eye Movement Desensitization and Reprocessing), developed by Francine Shapiro in 1988. It mystified and fascinated me. In brief, the client gathers a belief about the self, an emblematic memory, the corresponding emotion and whatever body sensation is associated with it, and holds all of them together. "Bilateral stimulation" in the form of side-to-side eye movement, rhythmic alternate-ear sound, or bilateral tapping, are applied, which facilitates processing. The result is that the original material loses its emotional charge and potency. It becomes memory rather than lived experience, and part of a narrative that is clearly located in the past.

As always, my first guinea pig was myself, and I found EMDR to be quite powerful in my own life as well. I worked with a skilled practitioner who combined it with art therapy, which for me was a winning combination and provided a rich access route. I quickly trained and became certified in it, and began passionately practicing EMDR. It proved to be tremendously effective as well as interesting to both myself and the client, although even now, I believe although much studied over these ensuing years and decades, we are not quite sure *why* it works.

At the time, in 1998, I was something of a lone wolf in my psychodynamic therapy community. Now, however, most of our field, including the arguably staid V.A., is friendly to EMDR. My experience with most of the modalities here described, and some are more "outside the box" than others, was that when they were new and unfamiliar to both colleagues and the client population, the therapist must be able to tolerate being different, and the sometimes-sideways glances of our colleagues. Coming from an attachment theory and psychodynamic clinical background and community, that was certainly a fact of life for me. Another pitch for solid and safe consultation.

As the trauma field progressed, and more and different methodologies emerged, EMDR stopped being my "go-to" approach, as there were others that seemed more a match to my personality, and to me more effective. Now, I almost never use EMDR, but I know from other practitioners that EMDR has continued to evolve in ways that are exciting, and increasingly effective. I still have great respect for it as a powerful trauma treatment, even though it is no longer my first choice. I do, however, have a handful of esteemed colleagues who do, and have continued to develop themselves as clinicians specializing in EMDR. Some have even found ways to administer it remotely during the Pandemic, when that is all we have. They have been a precious resource.

What I do continue to find useful is the practice of bringing together cognition (negative belief about the self), emotion, sensation and narrative and holding them all together. This is a key step in the EMDR protocol, before the bilateral stimulation is added. This intentional process, assembles the fragments of memory that are available, and also brings the respective disparate brain regions and brain functions into communication. Just holding still with that much material at once, can be powerful with developmental trauma clients especially with the added factor of a present and attentive, empathic other.

## SOMATIC THERAPY

I have always had a fascination with the body, and the mind/body interplay. And the body is often the battleground, or the stage where the neglect story metaphorically attempts to reveal itself. I have found somatic therapy approaches to particularly resonate with some of my neglect survivor clients who are very identified with their bodies, often athletes. Bill was one such. He was an ultradistance runner. A distance runner myself (although certainly not ultra!). I was still dumbfounded by his 100-mile treks through the night, up steep and muddy mountain trails – muscling on without sleep for days on end. It was a fitting description of life in his family, lonely, rugged, often painful, beset with using his own resources for navigating the course that would get him safely back; the mix of desolation and pride at doing it all himself.

Bill had no clear narrative, no coherent picture or story of his childhood. But I could ask him, and he could locate cues, the feeling he got on those long runs, including the long hours of solitary self-reflection or mind wandering. From the feelings he associated with his runs, we were able to assemble first at least the adjectives, if not the events, of his childhood. And as we did that, he became increasingly fluent in using verbal language, however, slowly. Little by little with practice, Bill came to understand that when he could identify no emotion or story, he might be able to locate a sensation somewhere in his body, that often contained valuable information. It might be an image, a memory fragment, or *something*. It was gratifying for him. And he also knew his brain was learning something important. I have never been so good at working with dreams. For me, the body has been the "royal road."

Similarly, Joel was a master rock climber. When he showed me pictures of the vertical walls of smooth granite that he scaled, preferring climbs that had never been attempted by anyone, I was stunned. He would have to pack in his 80 pounds of equipment to prepare the wall face, and then spend literally days making his way up. It was an incredible feat of strength and will, solitary much of the time. Weathering cold, sleeping on rock shelves or caves if he slept at all, reveling in the beauty. In the quiet of his solitude, he felt alive and content. He lived for those trips. The climbing became an access route for remembering the isolation, the quest to feel alive, and the deep wish to both demonstrate and be recognized for his extraordinary competence and accomplishment. He was aware that he had had a poverty of relationship in his life. He liked women but preferred those who were "very independent" so he could continue to be gone for a month at a time on his climbing trips, or in effect do what he wanted. He never imagined getting attached to a therapist. I don't know how we could have constructed the story so accurately without the entire through the climbing body.

Interestingly, when the Pandemic required that our sessions go to Zoom unfortunately, Joel's attentional challenge made it too difficult for us to continue meeting. He just found he could not stay present. He proposed, perhaps we continue our sessions walking in the park near my house. Between COVID safety and privacy concerns, we ultimately decided against it. But I trust he will be back.

Another client, Luisa, who would become gripped by anxious shame, and barrage herself with rhetorical questions, often questions of "why?" "Why did I wait so long to try and have babies?" "Why can't I just go to the gym?" "Why can't I just be happy with all the things I have?" The faster and the more insistent the litany of accusatory questions, the more hyper-aroused she would become. Soon she would be unbearably anxious. I would repeatedly interrupt her. "Luisa, these are all good questions. Any one of them alone could easily consume a whole session quite productively. Let's slow it down and take them one at a time." And I "taught" her to breathe. More accurately I taught her about the power of her breath, and of being mindful of it.

"Your inhale is sympathetic, it is stimulating. Your exhale is parasympathetic, it is calming. Breathe in on 6 counts, and out on 9 counts. Do that 10 times and see what you notice." She would quiet down, and we would go back and explore one question, and she might be able to slowly find her own answer and make use of it.

When a calmer, gentler, kinder, authentically curious part of herself asked the question. Luisa could feel not only relief from anxiety but also relief from shame. And she was able to recognize the frantic childhood feeling of casting about frenetically, lost, and terrified, with too many questions and no one to ask. She could then remember, there was no calm and steady, grounded other to turn to. She felt as if she could have drowned in that sea of not knowing what to do. She could readily re-constitute, relive that state, and often did.

Luisa also learned the steadying effect, of not only quieting her body but also of having a calm and interested other, listening to her. How dramatically and quickly that present other, changed her state. From that she was able to remember its opposite. She could then clearly remember, her mother's moods, Both her mother's anger and her absence. All from that simple intervention with breath. Besides simple interventions such as this one, there are whole formal treatment models designed to skillfully and methodically work with the body.

I studied Sensorimotor Psychotherapy (SP) and completed the entire formal training; and in a more piecemeal and intermittent way Peter Levine's Somatic Experiencing (SE) both very powerful. I found the training invaluable, and the work as well. Both trainings involved a lot of practicum, and opportunity to be the client and experience the work. In both modalities I experienced tremendous benefit, and I have seen the same with many clients. Formal trainings and workshops are readily accessible, although limited at the time of this writing, by the Pandemic. One of the great blessings of the Pandemic, however, has been a new wealth of webinars now available online. So even though the practicum is absent, or different, the theory and practical lectures are informative and wonderful.

More recently Ruth Lanius brought to my attention the work of Frank Corrigan, a brilliant neurobiologist, researcher and psychiatrist in Scotland, called Deep Brain Reorienting (DBR). The very first response to any trauma, not only in adults but also in all mammals, is the *orienting response*. This response is the core of Corrigan's method. The response happens so quickly that we are not aware of it. When a mother yanks the toddler quickly out of traffic, there is no time to think or feel. The brain registers the danger immediately and acts instantaneously out of survival necessity. The stimulus of the oncoming traffic goes to the most primitive area of the brain, the reptilian brain and the structures there called the Superior

Colliculus (SC), and the Periaqueductal gray (PAG). Without planning or emotion, that brain area orients the organism to the danger, and impels immediate action. With careful attention, when calling up a traumatic event, the tension in that area, the SC and the PAG, at the base of the skull at the back of the head, are discernible.

DBR has the client begin by recalling a present time upsetting experience, which even our neglect clients who have little memory would have access to. Recounting that will activate the orienting response. The client then tunes in to the sensation in that body area, and simply focuses on the body experience as it evolves and moves. The process is one of careful physiological tracking, without thought or emotion. Although I had heard of the orienting response before, I never would have imagined the power and the impact of using it as a point of entry for trauma processing.

Several sessions with Dr. Corrigan, have been profound for me, and made me want to learn this approach. In each case, I brought recent interpersonal material that I had had clearly disproportional feelings about and that I was struggling to shake. In each case, by the end of the session, the feeling had completely remitted, and I was visited by bits of memory that definitely correlated to it, and in one case even a new insight. It is my plan to add this work to my tool kit for neglect.

SP has a similar process called Sensorimotor Sequencing, also powerfully effective, which also tracks sensation in the body. The difference is that DBR targets specifically the orienting response, which is where the traumatic activation begins. As noted, Corrigan has coined the term "attachment shock" to describe the impact on the infant's nervous system of early attachment deficits, ruptures or other injuries. I believe any and all of these modalities to be beneficial to survivors of childhood neglect. And the more somatic skills the therapist has, the wider the range of clients and client difficulties, we can effectively and efficiently treat.

## NEUROFEEDBACK

What has become my go-to modality since I first learned of it in 2009, is Neurofeedback. It truly caught me unawares as I had reached an age and a point in my career, where I thought I was maybe "done" learning new approaches, and would kind of settle into what I already knew and work a little less hard. I found neurofeedback to be both irresistible, and the steepest learning curve I had encountered yet (until cheese-making!). I had grown up believing that I am not strong in science or math, and here I was faced with a wide world of neuroscience and technology: the brain and the computer. Oy vey. But I was hooked.

Neurofeedback is a form of biofeedback. The brain is not "zapped" as some people might think. It simply gets feedback about what it is already doing. It is a learning process, or a form of operant conditioning. As we are hard wired for positive re-enforcement, the brain learns to repeat activity that is "rewarded." The clinician after careful assessment sets the computer in what is estimated to be the desired frequency range for the client's targeted brain region; attaches electrodes to the corresponding area on the skull, and the client watches a computer game. During the game, when the requisite number of neurons are firing in the desired range, the computer registers a "reward" in the form of a sound or visual cue. The computer is in effect telling the brain "That is good, do that some more!" The positive reward, with sufficient practice, teaches the brain to default to this frequency. We are able to in effect "teach" the brain to fire at a level where the whole organism is calmer, or whatever would be optimal for that particular brain and body.

Fear of course is generally hyperarousal in the brain and nervous system. The brain, at least in certain areas, is firing too "high." Neglect often is a very anxious state as well, but depression and dissociation might also register as *hypo-arousal,* in which case, we need to train the brain "up." Different protocols target different brain areas, and some are designed to connect disconnected brain areas to each other.

Lanius' neurofeedback research includes MRI scans pre and post, to show how neurofeedback facilitates connectivity, and she describes dramatic treatment outcomes. That has been my experience as well. And when the story is absent or lacking it can generate material while also the increasing the ability to verbalize, enabling both processing of fear and making sense out of the story. Both support our ultimate task of reconstructing a coherent autobiographical narrative, and often without too much narrative to "go on."

Another advantage of neurofeedback is that during the actual neurofeedback processing, we don't talk. There is no need to revisit one's tired old story if one knows it, or search for something that can't readily be found. Many of our clients are tired of talking. To sink quietly into the perhaps confusing task of getting the computer to beep, without really knowing how we do it, might be a less taxing form of working. Best of all, it works more quickly than anything else I have studied and practiced. And a certain amount of mystery can make it something of a shared adventure.

Lanius is the world's top researcher on the neurobiology of trauma, and Sebern Fisher is the world's best on trauma and neurofeedback. They make a powerful duo as they research together. Much of their writing is in process. And those who search for research on neurofeedback will find it is sparse, because neurofeedback researchers largely have to find ways to scrape together their own funding, as most major research is paid for by big pharma, which is generally not interested in a process that helps people get off their meds. And they do. Still, there is much worth reading about neurofeedback.

I treated one severely traumatized woman with neurofeedback, for her chronic, unremitting, SUD 10 level migraine headaches. She was on three heavy medications all the time. After about a year of weekly neurofeedback, she was not only infinitely calmer and happier but also headache free and off all her medications. They never returned. For a while, she came for a periodic "tune-up" but not due to pain, rather just pre-emptively. Her neurologist was quite impressed.

Another woman, enraged and estranged from and not speaking to her mother for over six years, after six months of trauma processing with neurofeedback, went into therapy with her. They have since become best friends again. When couples therapy has been stalled, I have often proposed adding neurofeedback. Whether the problem was unremitting conflict, or sexual impasse, the neurofeedback did not "solve" it per se but changed the dynamic such as to be able to work with it differently, by ratcheting anger down to a point where partners could effectively speak and listen for example, or soften fear so as to enable an empathic ear.

I continue to learn constantly with neurofeedback. The literature steadily grows, and our little community continues to work to bring it into the mainstream. There is good data showing that neurofeedback provides effective treatment for addiction, ADD anxiety and depression, as well as trauma. And it is a highly rewarding pursuit for both therapist and client.

One drawback of neurofeedback is that besides the expense of training and much needed consultation, expensive equipment is required. So, if therapists themselves, are unable to become practitioners, locating good referrals so that resource is available to neglect survivor clients, can be a good addition to one's armamentarium. If possible, however, it is always preferable and more efficient, for the neurofeedback and psychotherapy to be localized within one therapist. The neurofeedback can elicit much material for psychotherapy, as well as transference. And utilizing the original attachment theory framework, the client's brain seems to be in resonance not only with the beeping computer but also with the therapist's brain. Perhaps that sounds a little magical, but it really does feel that way.

My father used to say, "Reading poetry in translation is like kissing a bride through a veil." That is rather how I feel if in a position to split the treatment in that way, and for the most part I won't do it anymore.

## ENTHEOGENS

In 2018, renowned author and professor at UC Berkeley Graduate School of Journalism, Michael Pollan published the blockbuster *How to Change Your Mind: The New Science of Psychedelics.* An accomplished, respected intellectual, certainly not the rabble that Richard Nixon blamed for the social ills of his era, put hallucinogenic drugs in the public eye, as a useful tool for mental health treatment. What was most publicized had been the research of treatment at UCLA with terminal cancer patients for their fear of death. I soon learned that significant and serious research is underway for the use of psychedelics in the treatment of trauma.

At the last few trauma conferences, and more general psychotherapy conferences there have been substantive presentations of successful trials with survivors of various kinds of trauma. Sessions are systematically prepared for with a therapist, and "guided," meaning the therapist both manages the dosage and is present with the client throughout the "journey" session, which is followed by multiple "integration" sessions, to powerful and accelerated effect. Currently, MDMA is in the final stages of the FDA approval process for clinical use with PTSD. And similar study is underway with Psilocybin (the active ingredient in hallucinogenic mushrooms), and LSD. Ketamine is already legal throughout the United States and in some other countries and is being successfully used for anxiety and other mental health complaints. In 2020,

*psilocybin* was legalized in Oregon. Results are hopeful, and again accelerated. The studies and research videos I saw presented in the conferences, showed the most rapid trauma processing and resolution I have ever seen. It is quite remarkable.

Graduate programs are already offering training in how to guide "entheogen," (hallucinogen) assisted psychotherapy sessions. We can look forward to these as a hopeful addition to our treatment options for developmental trauma and specifically neglect, in the not-too-distant future. I am intrigued, and although I don't see myself facilitating or guiding five and six-hour journey sessions, the therapists that do, seem to find them very rewarding.

## ATTACHMENT-ORIENTED PSYCHOTHERAPY

With all this being said, still there is no substitute for good, solid psychotherapy with a sensitive, highly conscious and well-attuned practitioner. Although talk therapy is not sufficient with neglect clients, it is equally essential. The core of the missing experiences is the failed, in-adequate, unpredictable primary caregiver. All that we do in the service of repairing that is foundational and ongoing.

Ruth Lanius in describing her neurofeedback trials with Developmental Trauma survivors, commented that she attributed the unusual zero drop-out rate they experienced, to the high quality of psychotherapy that accompanied the neurofeedback. She added, speaking about herself, "Neurofeedback forced me to be a better therapist, because of the volume of material it made available to work with." Whatever modalities we add, we must still continue to hone our craft, and again, maintain the best consultation we can. Which leads me to a last but certainly not least, "modality."

## CARE AND FEEDING OF YOUR MOST
## PRIZED INSTRUMENT

Therapist self-care, always essential, is particularly so with trauma, that often forces us to stare in the face of the most unbearable of human cruelty or failure. This work with neglect is in many ways particularly primitive. Because of its often-early developmental age, and often wordlessness, even more, is required of us. I often feel as if I need to run material through my own system, before it becomes digestible for the client, that it first appears in my body. However intimate and rewarding (although not always!) that is for us, it is also "metabolically expensive." I have also been struck by how particularly exhausting working remotely can be, especially with the added worry about technological disruptions/breakdowns. In addition to keeping ourselves safe and well from illness, we must stay mindful of keeping the instrument, our own selves, strong and regulated.

I remember it was 1995 when Charles Figley, a Vietnam veteran himself, coined the term "compassion fatigue." I promptly hopped on a plane to Florida to do a weekend workshop on it with him, having met and been startled by a very brilliant colleague who had truly burned herself out. It was no joke. She could not hear one more child's trauma story without going into dramatic trauma states, and turned to teaching art. It was frightening.

After 35 years I may be approaching balance. For a number of years, I had the hubris, and the grandiose belief that I could carry on with minimal sleep. I got away with it for quite a while, and I don't recommend it! We each have our own reservoirs of replenishment, and if we don't it is imperative to find them. We must also have the humility to know our limits, how much we can effectively do. Admittedly the social justice necessity and activity pulls on me to do more. It is a point of humility, as well as a responsibility to my neglected clients to keep myself well fed, rested, exercised, regulated and well balanced, and keep up with my own neurofeedback; so, my attention is reliable. I can always do better.

At the ripe age of 63, I discovered cheese making. Out of nowhere it bit me like a bug. Since I became interested in trauma, nothing had taken over my mind in that way. For a year, I read nothing but books about cheese, and I looked forward to every weekend when I could get back to stirring that vat. The science, art and history compelled me, and the process thrilled me. And also, somewhat unsettled me. I was busy *not* helping people. *Not* making a contribution to the world. Was that "OK?" I wasn't so sure.

Where I have landed, is that stirring the cheese vat calms me and regulates me. Learning the patience to wait many months or even years, for a cheese to be ready to eat; and many other metaphors and lessons, have value. I can make little packages and give them to my friends and family. But most significantly, making cheese makes me so happy. That does make me a better therapist.

## SUMMING UP AND WHAT TO DO

- Well-honed psychotherapy skills are essential for work with all clients, and most definitely neglect clients. Exquisitely attuned presence, mirroring, seeing and hearing, are the bones of our work.
- The therapist also needs a garage full of other tools with these clients, most specifically modalities that utilize other than cognitive and verbal means. And we need much more to flesh it out, and successfully carry out our task.
- EMDR, Somatic therapies, DBR and neurofeedback, are the ones I know best, but certainly not an exhaustive list. For each therapist, there will be an optimally "fitting" modality or modalities.
- Skilled and knowledgeable, trusted and regular consultation is imperative.
- Effective, restorative and consistent therapist self-care is an imperative component of our work.

## BIBLIOGRAPHY

Cohen, Michael P. *Neurofeedback 101: Rewiring the Brain for ADHD, Anxiety, Depression and Beyond (Without Medication)*. United States: Center for Brain Training, 2020.

Corrigan, Frank M., and Jessica Christie-Sands. "An Innate Brainstem Self-Other System Involving Orienting, Affective Responding, and Polyvalent Relational Seeking: Some Clinical Implications for a 'Deep Brain Reorienting' Trauma Psychotherapy Approach." *Medical Hypotheses* 136, no. 109502 (March 2020). https://doi.org/10.1016/j.mehy.2019.109502.

Fay, Deirdre. *Becoming Safely Embodied: A Guide to Organize Your Mind, Body and Heart to Feel Secure in the World*. New York: Morgan James, 2021.

Figley, Charles R. *Compassion Fatigue: Coping With Secondary Traumatic Stress Disorder in Those Who Treat the Traumatized. Brunner/Mazel Psychosocial Stress Series*. New York: Routledge, 1995.

Fisher, Sebern F. *Neurofeedback in the Treatment of Developmental Trauma: Calming the Fear-Driven Brain*. New York: W. W. Norton, 2014.

Levine, Peter A. *In an Unspoken Voice: How the Body Releases Trauma and Restores Goodness*. Berkeley, California: North Atlantic Books, 2010.

Ogden, Pat, and Janina Fisher. *Sensorimotor Psychotherapy: Interventions for Trauma and Attachment.* Norton Series on Interpersonal Neurobiology. New York: W. W. Norton, 2015.

Pollan, Michael. *How to Change Your Mind: What the New Science of Psychedelics Teaches Us About Consciousness, Dying, Addiction, Depression, and Transcendence.* New York: Penguin Press, 2018.

Ros, Tomas, Stefanie Enriquez-Geppert, Vadim Zotev, Kymberly D. Young, Guilherme Wood, Susan Whitfield-Gabrieli, Feng Wan, Patrik Vuilleumier, François Vialatte, and Dimitri Van De Ville. "Consensus on the Reporting and Experimental Design of Clinical and Cognitive-Behavioural Neurofeedback Studies (CRED-nf Checklist)." *Brain* 143, no. 6 (June 2020): 1674–1685. https://doi.org/10.1093/brain/awaa009.

Shapiro, Francine, and Margot Silk Forrest. *EMDR: The Breakthrough Therapy for Overcoming Anxiety, Stress, and Trauma.* New York: Basic Books, 2016.

Van der Kolk, Bessel A. *The Body Keeps the Score: Brain, Mind, and Body in the Healing of Trauma.* New York: Penguin Books, 2014.

Vernon, David, Ann Frick, and John Gruzelier. "Neurofeedback as a Treatment for ADHD: A Methodological Review With Implications for Future Research." *Journal of Neurotherapy* 8, no. 2 (May 2004): 53–82. https://doi.org/10.1300/J184v08n02_04.

White, Nancy E. "The Transformational Power of the Peniston Protocol: A Therapist's Experiences." *Journal of Neurotherapy* 12, no. 4 (December 2008): 261–265. https://doi.org/10.1080/10874200802502383.

# Chapter 11

# Conclusion

Reflecting on this work with survivors of the developmental trauma of neglect, I felt moved. It is a rather extraordinary privilege, like an incredible journey. With that thought a sudden flashbulb image emerged in my mind's eye: of a motley team: a small Siamese cat, flanked by two dogs: a sizeable yellow lab, and a big white bull terrier. The dogs loping through the snow on their long legs, the little cat lobbing, gracefully along, keeping up. A pop-up memory I have not had in years, of a movie I saw when I was probably about six. In it, by a series of errors and misunderstandings the three animals get separated from their human family. Together, somehow, they traverse two hundred and fifty miles of wild Canadian terrain, braving fierce winter weather, hunger, fatigue and treacherous large and small predators, to miraculously, reach their originally unknown destination. In full Disney glory the movie culminates in a dramatic, emotional reunion with the lost family. For me at six, without fully knowing why, it was a true tear-jerker. It is an awesome mystery how the memory may spontaneously surprise us with metaphors and fragments of sensory recall.

We may look from the outside, like an odd pair, an unlikely partnership. And a homecoming of sorts is what our neglect clients may or may not know that they long for. It may not explicitly turn out to be the loving family of origin, but rather perhaps peace about the not so loving family. It may be coming" home" to a more coherent sense of self; relief from the chronic gnawing emptiness of disconnection, and the bodily and emotional relief of feeling connected to someone, and perhaps more integrated. It really is as incredible as Disney's story, (which is a well-crafted work of fiction).

Sometimes the journey is long, rather comparable to 250 miles for a small Siamese. Thinking it through in more detail, my client "Jim" whose story lopes in and out through these chapters has been with me nearly three decades. That skinny kid I first met, was in his early late twenties and just turned 60. In our journey, some of the treacherous predators, were our experience of each other, which we also miraculously survived.

Jim adventurously accompanied me through the tasting menu of serial modalities, and has been an expressive living and verbal responder about their comparative efficacy, at least their efficacy for him. Of course, some of the "magic" is harder for him to see, most decidedly in his relatedness, which sometimes moves me to tears. Yes, sometimes it takes that long. The reader may find a decades long treatment horrifying or simply impractical. I am sure if we had had neurofeedback thirty years ago, it would have shaved off at least a decade or two. And nonetheless, replicating early development, is not quick. It absolutely does *not* always take this long. Admittedly I do have immense hope that the psychedelics will be approved soon for clinical use. To me they show great promise, and the way they work in the brain, which is beyond the scope of this book, seems most suitable for the brain disconnected by neglect.

Jim responded more than generously when I asked if I might write about bits and pieces of our story. He was not only willing but also excited to be of help to others. I hesitantly asked, "Even the infamous 'incident?" He did not miss a beat in responding, "Absolutely!" He looks for any opportunity to "reciprocate" to me, jumping at the chance to provide for example tech support, with the inevitable tech challenges of this Pandemic.

Jim can now express gratitude that I hung in with him all these years, through our snow and porcupines, and bears. And he can express gratitude for the neurofeedback, which has been wondrous for him, but also all the other modalities in our multivariate approach. He appreciates that I was willing to be the oddball in town, who used the various "new-fangled" approaches that seemed like snake oil to the larger community. It is not atypical, for someone like Jim to be in no hurry to leave the relationship. With much of his family now deceased, I am rather like family. We can only say "who would have thunk it?" And even all the cheese in the world can't beat that.

Neglect has been hidden in shadow for so long. As we drag it into view, we can see the many tentacles it has. It is intimately tied to incident and shock trauma. Under parents' attentive eyes, at least some of the terror that children experience would be noticed, and even stopped, Nonetheless, however, in and of itself, without an additional overt trauma, to see and identify that to be unseen and not known or understood, is a profound and "under-rated" devastation is even more uncanny and awesome to our clients. We are bringing what was truly invisible, even to them, into the bright light of day. They can't imagine that they matter that much.

Amy Tan, in her deeply sensitive memoir simply and profoundly states, that loneliness is not about being alone. Rather, it is about not being understood. Providing this experience, which our clients generally do not even know is missing, can be not only unimaginable, but also immeasurably powerful. When I first started therapy at the age of 23, I believed I had to start the relationship anew in each session. I could not imagine that another person might hold me in mind, that I might exist when I was not in her sight. And when she even remembered what I told her, it bordered on astonishing. My parents never knew the names of my few friends, and my father always referred to my first boyfriend, who I had for seven years, as "that man." It was astonishing that my therapist somehow held my whole life with me.

Understanding, or working at understanding also often involves, translating the symptoms: the body expressions, the behaviors, the re-enactments, the relationship patterns, the often-confounding presence or absence of emotion, the self-destructive habits, to help them transform all this mess into narrative. All of this makes us very special. We have to earn this spot, over and over again. It also makes us unique in our interest. "Who would care that much to make a project of understanding *me*?"

Some of our clients have children. Often those kids are a living symbol and ongoing reminder of why it is important to do their work, and be different from their own parents. That has always been an inspiration and a motivator for me. And often these clients only begin to comprehend the impact of their own experience, when we use the example of their own child going through something even vaguely comparable. Then they begin to get it. Yes, part of our task and a blessed by-product of our work, is breaking the intergenerational chain. As a child of two highly traumatized parents, I feel both a deep sense of responsibility and also a profound feeling of privilege, even pride, to be able to participate in the world in that way.

Another of the insidious tentacles of neglect, is the vast and complex web of social justice. Poverty, race, war, parental addiction; failures of health care, child care and education, make it possible or even inevitable, for children to be forgotten and harmed. How many children are left to fend for themselves, or are forgotten, because their parents have to work night and day, or are in jail, or die of failed or lacking health care like my father's mother when he was too young? And what about all those children separated from parents at the border? The reach of these tentacles is massive. I don't include this to overwhelm, but rather because not to at least acknowledge it, would seem neglectful at best. It also lends humility to our work. Neither to under nor over-estimate, what we can do. The function or dysfunction in the larger environment, or the behavior of a prevailing political system can be the inescapable replica of all sorts of abuse and neglect. And can perpetuate it. Sadly, singlehandedly we can neither control nor prevent it, (and often are hard pressed to manage our own feelings about it!) I know I am committed to doing all I can, and must not have the hubris or grandiosity to overestimate what that might be. We must do our best, sometimes for protracted periods of time, to help our clients regulate their reactivity, or even their news consumption. None of this is easy.

The attachment bond is the centerpiece of our work. The profound, pervasive and persistent dysregulations of brain and body stem back to that. An integrative approach that incorporates a panoply and a menu of interventions and access routes, is essential. As long as we remember, that the functions of presence, mirroring, seeing, believing and tracking, are most fundamental. At that, we must never waver. And we won't get it perfectly of course.

For me the study of the brain, and the inclusion of the brain in this work are key. Attachment and the body, emotion, sensation and regulation, all begin to come together and make sense in this endlessly fascinating and miraculous organ.

When Bessel van der Kolk first started talking about the brain in the early 1990s, I was compelled and cowed. Being one of those many girls of my generation that early on were led to believe that girls are good in reading and writing and stupid in math and science, I was swimming upstream to learn about it. But seeing how normalizing and helpful it was to clients when I made a poster-sized replica of van der Kolk's scans of the brain in a trauma state, made it worthwhile to continue the swim. The appearance of Jaak Panksepp's book Affective Neuroscience in 1998, was my introduction to the underpinnings of emotion in the brain, body and nervous system, so relevant to everything we do with this population, and any clients really.

We now know so much more about the brain, most significantly that the brain is plastic, neurogenesis is possible, the brain can grow, heal and regenerate itself I certainly did not learn that in graduate school. It definitely changes how we can think about our task, and what our clients imagine they can hope for.

I am grateful to have learned about neurofeedback in 2009 and to have had the opportunity to study and practice it ever since. It frustrates me that such a powerful and effective modality does not yet reach the mainstream; and also, is so expensive for clinicians to both learn and then buy equipment to practice. So, its use is still limited and inaccessible to the less privileged. Nonetheless, I encourage readers to learn about it and at the very least find local practitioners for referrals.

As of this writing, we are still in the midst of the Pandemic of 2020: COVID 19, which has already spanned nearly a year. It has been tragic to watch how many have lost their lives, livelihoods, sometimes both. I have been blessedly fortunate, that all of my loved ones have stayed well, that my City has been well led, and has fared relatively well; and that I have been able to continue my work with most clients via Zoom.

Just as our three furry journeyers ate things on their journey they would not have considered even tasting when in their comfy home; so am I learning about things I never could have imagined, as have my clients. Jim, gained verbal fluency that he had never had before in therapy, because we had always had other much more "interesting" and helpful methodologies.

Jackie was encouraged and inspired to discover that the gains she had achieved in self-regulation from the neurofeedback, held and were sustained; and enabled her to make the most of the challenges of Lockdown. And we all learned something about our primary attachments.

I also never imagined I would work from home. Zoom made me visible and human in a new way, even if only in the one room of my house that showed up on the screen. If shame is about hiding, I was now a little bit more exposed. And like Miss Wiesjahn in the grocery store when I was six, I became more like my clients just as Miss Wiesjahn was really just a person like me. All of this bears on the relationship. And somehow, I think I feel calmer, more myself and more accessible.

One of the many, many losses of the Pandemic, has been the innumerable cancellations. Not only our clinical conferences where we get to see each other. The arts have been tragically decimated by the end to public gatherings. Concerts, museums, dance performances, theater, even movies have been forced to go remote. Education has been slammed, with even young children forced to stay home and look at a screen, if they even have one, not to mention graduate programs. And recreational travel has screeched to a stop, with many long-anticipated vacations, being canceled generating huge disappointment.

For our neglect clients, waiting is next to unbearable. This is a signature complaint. Feeling powerless about having any impact, and hard pressed to believe they exist in anyone's mind, they don't expect to be remembered, or that the other will ultimately return. Missing out on events and trips and all the other many cancellations are a terrible traumatic reminder.

A vital part of our task is to be relentless hope mongers, to routinely as my father instructed (and also did), hit every sold-out concert. I repeatedly tell my clients, "it is part of my job to hold the hope, to carry the hope when you can't. I can do that."

## BIBLIOGRAPHY

Markle, Fletcher. *The Incredible Journey*. Burbank, California: Walt Disney Productions, 1963.

Panksepp, Jaak. *Affective Neuroscience: The Foundations of Human and Animal Emotions. Series in Affective Science.* New York: Oxford University Press, 1998.

Tan, Amy. *Where the Past Begins: A Writer's Memoir.* New York: ECCO, 2017.

# Index

For Product Safety Concerns and Information please contact our EU
representative GPSR@taylorandfrancis.com
Taylor & Francis Verlag GmbH, Kaufingerstraße 24, 80331 München, Germany

www.ingramcontent.com/pod-product-compliance
Ingram Content Group UK Ltd.
Pitfield, Milton Keynes, MK11 3LW, UK
UKHW021448080625
459435UK00012B/408